OWN YOUR AWKWARD

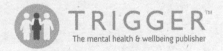

TRIGGER™

The mental health & wellbeing publisher

About the Author

Michelle Morgan is a leading voice in mental health and a proud Ambassador for Mental Health First Aid England. In 2016 Michelle experienced burnout, anxiety and depression. She views her mental health challenges as both a burden and a blessing; from a terrible time, good things came.

Michelle is an Mindfulness-Based Cognitive Therapy (MBCT) Instructor, an international speaker and corporate trainer (clients include Facebook, HSBC, Pukka Herbs, The Prime Minister's Office, Red Bull and Good Energy). She is also the Founder of Pjoys – PJs with Purpose, and Co-founder of Livity, a creative business that works with brands and the next generation to "build the future better".

Her work has been widely lauded: she is the recipient of the Queen's Award for Enterprise and EY Entrepreneur of the Year Award, and has been invited to join the Society of Leadership Fellows at St George's House, Windsor Castle.

She lives in London with her husband, artist Remi Rough, their daughter Lili and dog Teddy. Connect with her at www.michellemorgan.uk and www.ownyourawkward.com. Find her on Instagram @michellemorgan.uk and on Twitter @michellemorgan.

OWN YOUR AWKWARD

How to Have Better and Braver Conversations
About Our Mental Health

Michelle Morgan

Foreword by Simon Blake OBE
CEO Mental Health First Aid England

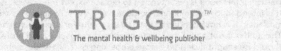

TRIGGER™
The mental health & wellbeing publisher

This edition published in 2023 by Trigger Publishing
An imprint of Shaw Callaghan Ltd

UK Office
The Stanley Building
7 Pancras Square
Kings Cross
London N1C 4AG

US Office
On Point Executive Center, Inc
3030 N Rocky Point Drive W
Suite 150
Tampa, FL 33607
www.triggerhub.org

Text Copyright © 2021 Michelle Morgan
First published by Welbeck Balance in 2021

A CIP catalogue record for this book is available upon request from the British Library

World excluding USA, Canada & Philippines: Extract from: *A Mindfulness Guide
for the Frazzled* by Copyright © Ruby Wax 2016, published by Penguin Life 2016.
Reprinted by permission of Penguin Books Limited.

USA, Canada & Philippines: Excerpt from *A Mindfulness Guide for the
Frazzled* by Ruby Wax reprinted by permission of Peters Fraser & Dunlop
(www.petersfraserdunlop.com) on behalf of Ruby Wax.

ISBN: 978-1-83796-292-1
Ebook ISBN: 978-1-83796-293-8

Cover design by Steve Williams
Cover image by Remi Rough
Typeset by Lapiz Digital Services

For my loves Remi and Lili.

In memory of Dave Moore.

Foreword

Being human means having a wide range of feelings, thoughts and experiences. Joyful ones, difficult ones and everything in between. Yet society has taught us from a really young age that mental health is not something we talk about openly – with confidence, sensitivity, compassion and kindness.

Too many of us grew up learning that mental health conversations are off limits and mental illness is frightening. While we are, thankfully, seeing a slow shift as the next generation talk more openly about their mental health, stigma and silence still remain; perhaps especially so for those of us born in the last century.

All of us will be touched either directly or indirectly by poor mental health or mental illness at some point in our lives. By developing our understanding around mental health we can both protect and nourish our own wellbeing, and spot the signs of poor mental health in others, offering support and signposting to professional help.

In doing so we can literally change – and ultimately save – lives.

This book reminds us that we have the power to break the silence. We have the power to replace misinformation with accurate information, and we have the power to replace stigma, silence and fear with compassion, empathy for others, self-love and non-judgemental support.

Michelle is one of a growing number of people who have generously chosen to share their story and experience, with the aim of creating the kinder and more compassionate world we hope for. She leads by example and demonstrates that you don't have to be perfect to take a deep breath and get started.

In *Own Your Awkward* you will find wisdom and insights from a collection of voices, as well as practical tools, frameworks and mantras to inspire, educate and encourage reflection. You will also find practical exercises to help you develop insight into your feelings – especially the awkward ones, build "conversation courage" and practical skills.

Conversations about mental health – much like riding a bike, driving a car or, in fact, virtually everything in life – *do* get easier with practice.

As we grow up, far too many of us learn to be awkward and embarrassed. The sad truth is that we often spent more time at school learning "helpful" facts (which turn out not to be that helpful after all) than we did learning to listen, to care, and have good, quality conversations. And that is still true for children and young people growing up now – in an age when we can Google everything.

I often joke that I wish I could listen and ooze empathy and care without saying a word even half as well as my dog, Dolly, does. Truth is, I wish we all could.

We may never develop Dolly's levels of comfort with just sitting with the silence, saying nothing and letting another person talk and sometimes cry. However, we can all – one conversation at a time – create a more open culture where we value mental health, where we can talk about it and where we can get help and support when we need it.

In a world that still stigmatizes mental health and that can prevent us talking about how we really feel and really listening to how others feel, I am grateful to Michelle for writing this book. I know it has been a labour of love.

And I want to say thank you to you for buying this book. I hope it will inspire you to Own Your Awkward and do all you can each day to reduce unhelpful and damaging stigma.

Simon Blake OBE
Chief Executive, Mental Health First Aid England

Contents

Introduction

"It's a bit awkward when you talk about your mental health Michelle." Crushing, embarrassing, silencing and, just like that, as a result of one careless and stigmatizing remark I stepped out of Livity, the youth-led creative studio and consultancy I had co-founded 16 years earlier, under a cloud of immense shame and an even greater sense of self-loathing than I was already experiencing, communicated through a mysterious, vague and vanilla, almost chipper-sounding message to my dear work family. Just look at all those optimistic and cheerful exclamation marks in this note:

Hi Livity Fam,

I hope you're all having a brilliant start to 2017!

It's going to be a good one, we have a great plan, great people and a great purpose. Here's to a great year!

I wanted to let you know that I will be out of the office for a short while addressing some health matters. I'll be staying connected to the biz remotely for the next few weeks and then will be offline for a bit concentrating on making a full and speedy recovery.

I'll be really looking forward to catching up with you all soon!

Big love, Meesh x

The words that make up that note are the mask of mental illness, my mental illness. It's amazing how long we can pretend to be "just fine" when the truth is, we're really not fine at all. What I was actually experiencing was a violent physical and mental burnout, which had fast developed into a terrifying combination of yet undiagnosed clinical depression and anxiety. I wrote to the team, utterly believing that I'd be back in my role and the business in next to no time.

"I'll be really looking forward to catching up with you all soon!" In fact, I never returned to the day-to-day running of Livity.

IT'S *NOT* AWKWARD!

On the other side of that terrible time, as a business leader and entrepreneur, an ambassador and instructor for Mental Health First Aid (MHFA) England, a Mindfulness-Based Cognitive Therapy instructor, and as a wife, mother, daughter, sister, friend, co-worker and woman, I've now shared my experience of burnout, depression and anxiety hundreds of times, to thousands of people. Sometimes just to one person, often to teams, groups and networks of people, and also on stage, usually wearing a pair of pyjamas (more about *that* later) to audiences of hundreds and what I have discovered is this … It's not actually that awkward talking about mental health. REPEAT IN JOYFUL SHOUTY CAPS, IT'S NOT AWKWARD!

IT *IS* AWKWARD!

Hmm, WAIT! REWIND. Well, okay, maybe it is *sometimes* awkward. Err, well actually, perhaps it is awkward *most times* when we talk about mental health. But, really, how long does it stay awkward? At this stage of my life, with everything I have experienced and learned, it's only usually awkward for a few minutes. That moment when either I'm about to tell you (or a whole bunch of people) about my mental health or I'm going to ask you about yours. That moment when I just don't know how the words are going to land with you if I tell you about mine or how you are going to respond if I ask you how you are feeling or if everything is okay. That moment when my head is telling me this is potentially going to be awkward and difficult, and maybe it would be best to retreat as fast as possible and not utter a word. It is the moment I am feeling a rise in stress, anxious, with a dry mouth, racing heart, sweaty palms and, perhaps, even a sense of mild, but escalating panic in my mind and my body, which despite being natural mental and physical responses, as we'll explore in Chapter 3 of this book, are still pretty horrible and confusing.

Worried About Offering Help

If I'm thinking about offering help to someone, if I want to ask them if they are okay or check in with them about their mental health, I'm maybe worrying about how they'll feel if I say those words "mental health" or mention "feelings" and "wellbeing" even. I might be concerned that I could make the person *feel* worse, *make* things worse. Or perhaps I've got it wrong, maybe they're okay and it would be embarrassing for me and for them to suggest something isn't right. I'm thinking, what if I fluster or trip up over my words? What if I go blank? What if I use the wrong words? I'm scared of offending them or making assumptions that are just not true or accurate. I'm asking myself who the heck am I to assume anything about anyone's feelings and situations? And, worst of all, what if something *is* wrong and they start telling me about it, what then? What will I say? How will I be able to fix it? I seem to have got myself into a right old mess, before I've even opened my mouth. I start thinking, maybe I should just keep quiet, I'll sit tight, move on, say nothing, don't upset the apple cart. I'm thinking this is all a bit awkward.

Does all that sound familiar? It is so easily and often the unhelpful narrative in our heads.

Worried About Asking for Help

On the flip side, if I'm struggling with *my* mental health and wellbeing, I'm fragile. I'll likely be experiencing embarrassment, shame and, possibly, a ton of self-loathing even. I probably don't know where to start a conversation about how I'm feeling, how to say it, when to say it? I'm imagining all the different and devastating responses I may receive, unable to imagine the possibility of a positive and caring one. I might not be aware of it, but I'm already feeling judged. I'm feeling silly, stupid and pathetic. The unhelpful "What ifs?" are coming thick and fast. The feeling of being a burden may be intensifying because, crikey, I really don't want to add my woes to someone else's life, they've probably got enough on their plate without me becoming a weight of responsibility.

This, of course, is all adding to how bad I'm feeling already, so perhaps I can reduce my pain by taking my head out of these thoughts of asking for help. Perhaps I'd be better to just get on with life, as I was, and not talk about it. To be honest, I'm thinking this is all a bit awkward.

Better and Braver Conversations

You see what I've discovered and, look, it's taken a very long time and a bucket-load of pain and support to get there, is that if you can just push on through those few awkward seconds and minutes, push on through the fear and uncertainty of how someone is going to respond, whether you're offering help or asking for help, more often than not, it's a good thing, a helpful thing, maybe even a lifesaving thing (really), to be able to talk honestly about how you are feeling in both your body and mind.

While I may still not always have a constant and confident frame of mind, by transforming that feeling of panic into power, I believe I build deeper and more meaningful relationships with people, much more quickly, by openly talking about my own mental health and that of others. I know, because people have told me that I've encouraged and assisted them toward help, and I've most certainly supported my own recovery and ongoing mental health management, by having better and braver conversations. Because, you see, when I'm honest about my mental health, I connect with other humans who then often find it easier to talk about their own experiences. I feel less alone, they feel less alone. It's a win/win. But yes, okay, I concede, it *is* awkward and that's why we are here, to learn how to face that awkward moment and embrace it. Own it!

A Fear of Mental Illness

Early beliefs about the causes of mental ill-health included spiritual and demonic possession, and these remain in some cultures even today ... Whaaaat? Yes, and the stereotypical view of mental illness continues to rage, with the misguided belief that people with mental ill-health are dangerous, aggressive and violent to others, when the truth is they are likely to be of more harm to themselves than anyone else, sometimes with the most tragic of outcomes. These beliefs are inflamed and reinforced through what we watch, listen to and read. The media, literary and entertainment industries, in their own ways, report or tell stories of people experiencing mental illness in the most dangerous, criminal and evil of ways, sinister wrong 'uns, unable to live regular, fulfilled lives and very rarely with any positive outcomes. Great and gripping viewing, reading and listening, perhaps, but stigmatizing and unhelpful for both those who want to offer help and ask for help, fuelling fear and misunderstanding and fast-tracking the decision to ask for or offer support into the "avoidance bucket". Too difficult, too risky and yep, you've got it, too awkward to talk about.

Transforming Panic into Power

This book is about Owning Your Awkward in order to get comfy having uncomfy conversations about mental health. I've written it to change the narrative – to turn the silence and stigma I experienced into a very loud klaxon, and to share my story of mental ill-health with even greater numbers of people. I'm determined to continue playing my part in smashing the stigmas around poor mental health and give you the confidence and capability to play your part. I'm not solely here to share my story, I'm here to share what I've learned. I'm going to help you understand why that fear and difficulty emerges in those awkward moments and help you transform them into your power. Reality check – I'm not promising you a Super Power. I do believe, though, that I can help you tap into your innate skills, compassion and courage, and strengthen and build them so that you can unleash the power of communication that you naturally possess to start a conversation. Even more than that, I'm Owning MY Awkward so that you can own YOURS.

GETTING TO KNOW YOU

I've found myself wondering about you – who you are and why you are reading this book. I wonder what you are hoping for, expecting or perhaps are simply interested in. It's highly likely you are here because you want to feel more confident offering support to someone you think or know is experiencing mental health issues and that's a beautiful and generous place to start. Perhaps you want to take the brave step of learning how to ask for help and support for yourself, or maybe you are simply connecting and enjoying the idea of Own Your Awkward and curious to know more. I love it when people immediately "get" the idea just from those three words … Whatever your reason for picking up this book, please just stop for a moment and give yourself a great big, excruciatingly awkward, pat on the back.

Why? Because you are taking action. You are here reading or listening because you are open to ideas and to developing your ability to talk more easily and often about mental health. And this book is not only about offering and asking for help, it's about understanding and supporting your own mental health in order to be better placed to support others – and that's not just a nice added bonus, it's critical. What I've learned about mental health is that whether you're offering help, asking for help or helping yourself, you can't really do or be great at one, without embracing the other two.

An Acknowledgement of Privilege

In many ways my story and experience of mental illness is told from a place of privilege as a white British, cisgender woman. I'm aware that there are people with far greater challenges and vulnerabilities with both their mental health and their general circumstances and backgrounds, and I'm incredibly grateful for the support I had around me and the provisions I had access to. Without both, I'm not sure what the outcome might have been – not good I suspect, not good at all.

Nonetheless, it's not a competition. It was a truly terrible and terrifying time, the lowest of lows I've ever experienced for a sustained amount of time, and the most fragile and broken I have ever felt. I've found along the way that sharing my story connects and helps others, and my mantra is that if sharing my story helps just one person, then it was worth sharing and I encourage the same of you. Whatever your story of mental health, please know that it's worth telling and sharing. Even if it doesn't feel as "good" or "bad" to you as someone else's, doesn't mean it is any less important and it really might connect and help another person. Imagine that! Value yourself and your story.

HOW TO USE THIS BOOK

Asking for help, offering help and helping ourselves are inextricably linked, and you will boost your ability to do them all more confidently by learning to understand, manage and Own Your Awkward. I'm dedicated to showing you how and why. Here's our roadmap through this book:

1. My story and how it led me to my new purpose.
2. Understanding mental health and recognizing that we all have it.
3. Why we are wired to panic and feel awkward and what we can do about it.
4. Learn the Four Steps To Owning Your Awkward.
5. The SENSE framework that will help you Own Your Awkward to help others.
6. How to listen – really listen – and the extraordinary power of the pause.
7. The BRAVE framework that will help you Own Your Awkward to ask for help.
8. Self-care is not selfish! Why taking care of yourself is an essential part of helping others.

9. The M-Plan – inspiration and ideas for self-care.
10. Celebrating awkward.

The book ends with a reference section of common mental health conditions, which will further cultivate your confidence, as well as signposting you to further resources.

It's worth noting that there are chunks and chapters that, if missed and unread, might, perhaps, mean a missed lesson or lightbulb moment even – so enjoy this reading journey, as best you can, logically and directly from A to B (Chapters 1 to 10). Mostly, though please, enjoy reading the book in whatever way best suits you; if you are a dipper or a skimmer, that's okay. We are all different, a human fact to be celebrated.

With a Little Help from My Friends

This book is not all me, me, me. I've shared the stories, experiences and wisdom of a bunch of generous pals, peers and professionals who I've connected with in a variety of ways on my journey to recovery and my "what next" in life. Essentially, I've done one of the things that I still find challenging and that is to ask for help – one of the main messages of this book. I thought I'd better lead by example! Believe me, if I can push through the awkward and ask for help, so can you – stick with me to find out how.

Alongside my awkward tales, we'll get a glimpse into how other people have experienced their own awkward moments – the successes, the failures and how they have learned to Own Their Awkward. When we arrive at The M-Plan in Chapter 9, you'll find many of them have also shared their self-care (ouch, there's that uncomfy word again) practices. This book is a way to share, amplify and pass on the things that have worked for me and for others and that you can pass on and use yourself. After all, sharing is caring.

My story and the stories shared in this book are not recommendations for how to diagnose or treat mental ill-health. Rather, they are experiences and insights shared in the spirit of generosity to help make it easier for others to become aware of and talk about both their own, and other people's, mental health; to normalize it, perhaps create a moment of connection and recognition for someone or, at the very least, just to be able to be more open and honest about how we are feeling.

But it's not simply storytelling; I've packed this book with what I believe are frameworks and formulas worth testing and giving a go. Stories to help you connect, logic to help you act and a little magic to inspire and encourage you along the way.

Try This ...

I've always believed in learning by doing and so have woven some simple, interactive and non-obligatory Try This ... exercises into each chapter. They are there to bring important points to life, to land key messages and help you understand yourself and others better. As you respond to and reflect on each exercise, you might want to have a notebook or journal at hand, or use the notes app on your phone. Or you may simply want to ponder each one silently or discuss them with someone else. Experiment and find the best way for you.

What This Book is Not Here to Do

This book won't make you a mental health professional (if you are not already one). It won't teach you to diagnose or treat people with mental health issues – that's not your job, nor the job of this book. The more formal information I share has been either checked or compiled by mental health professionals, for whom I have huge respect, or comes from recognized mental health organizations. It is included to help give context and knowledge (which will give you more confidence) and support the frameworks I have created for starting conversations. The frameworks are just that – support for *starting* conversations and then *signposting* people toward the right kind of help or assisting you in seeking it out for yourself.

Keeping Safe

While I hope that this book makes you feel positive and reassured, and even makes you smile along the way, I'm aware that it might also bring up difficult, sad, confusing or even surprising feelings too. Remember, it's okay to not feel okay, but it's also my belief that it's not okay to continually not be okay. If you notice that the book is triggering difficult thoughts and feelings, it's important to ask for help, especially if any distressing feelings seem to be hanging around or escalating. On page 265 you'll find resources and signposting to support you, or think about a friend, family member or co-worker you trust and have a (beautifully awkward) conversation with them.

THE CORNERSTONES OF AWKWARD CONVERSATIONS

CONFIDENCE | CAPABILITY | COMMUNICATION COMPASSION

No one should ever feel so awkward talking about mental health that it actually stops them from talking about it. To help make mental health an everyday conversation and to help you Own Your Awkward, I've identified four attributes that I believe to be the cornerstones to having easier and better, even if still a little uncomfortable, conversations about mental health. We're here to get comfy with the uncomfy and the cornerstones provide solid foundations for taking the steps to Owning Your Awkward, supporting you through any discomfort (and there will be some!), alongside the stories, frameworks, ideas, information, logic and, I hope, a whole lot of magic, you will find in this book.

1. Confidence

My intention is to give you a greater sense of confidence, by providing you with a greater level of understanding of mental health in an accessible and actionable way. I'm not going to overwhelm you with in-depth details and science; let's be clear, I'm not a scientist – but I will share, with the help of some actual brilliant mental health professionals and organizations, useful and practical references to help bring to life elements of how our marvellous, yet ever so mysterious and somewhat complex, minds work, thrive or sometimes wobble and break, and how that impacts our ability to have confident conversations about mental health, whether asking for help or offering it.

When I lead mental health awareness and training sessions, I witness the simple, yet powerful, benefits and confidence boost that people get from a little more know-how about both the broad topic of mental health and issues associated with it and how to talk about it. Knowledge is not only power, it's confidence! So, at the end of the book, compiled with the help of the team at HelloSelf, a UK-based platform providing access to clinical psychologists, and the organization that has supported me with my mental ill-health, you'll find introductory explanations and definitions of some of the most common diagnosable mental illnesses and disorders.

2. Capability

A bit like sitting down to write this book, page by page, chapter by chapter, each time a blank page is the painful, yet inevitable starting point. Conversations about mental health can be similar. A metaphorical blank page, a silence, a "where to start?", a sense of awkwardness. Sometimes the best way is just to get going, to begin, to know that action, taking a deep breath and going for it, as opposed to not giving it a go and perhaps never knowing what might have been, is courageous. With this book you can prepare, practise and expand your skills and sense of capability. I'm here to help you feel less stuck on the blank page and in the deafening silence that comes in advance of a tricky or nerve-racking conversation.

The frameworks I've created provide tangible starting points, places to jump off from and into a conversation and to keep coming back to, checking in with and trying out aspects of, in different ways. I hope in their simplicity they feel mighty and memorable. BRAVE: How to ask for help and SENSE: How to offer help, will expand your capability and boost your confidence. The Four Steps To Owning Your Awkward is a tool you can take and use way beyond the subject of mental health. You'll be better equipped to talk about your own and other people's mental health, and you'll have a new set of valuable assets to keep to hand in your toolkit/handbag/briefcase/backpack (select and delete as you wish) of metaphorical aids.

3. Communication

Own Your Awkward is a call to action, a manifesto and shift in mindset that will change how you and, I hope, others think, feel, do and communicate when poor mental health presents itself in some shape or form, all whilst recognizing, as we'll learn, that these shapes and forms can be wildly different and varied from one another. Because when we take ownership of those awkward moments, whether we're about to tell someone about *our* mental health or ask someone about *theirs*, we'll find that, with a little care and thought, it doesn't actually have to be that difficult and it can even be, at the very least, a welcome relief and release and, at the very most, an absolute life-enhancing, joyful and freeing experience. The skill and the success we hope for is in *how* we communicate, both verbally and physically. It's as much about language and listening as it is about the how, when and where. Together, we'll learn how to maximize our communication skills, whether in a one-to-one setting or through the spirit of imparting this rallying cry of Own Your Awkward to our families, friends, co-workers and communities.

4. Compassion

What you have in this book and idea of Owning Your Awkward, I sincerely hope, is a truly human and compassionate approach to understanding mental health and talking about it more comfortably and easily. Yes, we are going to work on how we become comfortable feeling uncomfortable, but uncomfortable doesn't mean unkind, nor crass – the conversations we have will be led with compassion and kindness and the frequent reminders of why we are here, deep somewhere in the pages of this awkward book. After all, we're here to help others, support those who need it and, perhaps, a little more difficult to admit, we're also here to support ourselves. View this book as quite simply a compassionate conversation starter. Most challenging of all will be the compassion that I invite you to bring to yourself when we step into the topic of self-care. I can feel your shudder as I write the word, but don't worry as my M-Plan (see Chapter 9) is going to change how you see and feel about the S-C word!

The Compassion starts here ... I'm going to be with you, every awkward step of the way through this book, because by Owning My Awkward I hope to successfully help you to take ownership of yours and then maybe you will help others take ownership of theirs.

GIVING LESS OF YOURSELF TO GIVE MORE

Before my burnout and over the first 16 years of co-founding and running Livity, I tried my best to lead with compassion. Of course, it's important to say that it wasn't always a success. I was, however, connected in some emotional way to most, if not all, of the people who came through our doors. I was often, though not always, an easy person to talk to. On reflection, and this feels hard to write, I'd spend and give far more of my time supporting people in and around the business than was always realistic or appropriate. I would often drop into solution-finding, fixing, advising and even, some might say, "saving" mode. Often finding myself in scenarios that I wasn't wholly equipped or experienced to support with, and highly likely for too long, I carried a huge weight of responsibility on my shoulders, and in my head and heart, and in some ways a feeling of obligation to go the extra mile and hours to help and support those who needed it.

The consequence of this was that I spent less time with my husband, Remi, and daughter, Lili. Time I'll never have back. You simply can't be in two places at once and trying to leave the Livity office sometimes felt almost impossible, driven by the concern of letting people down, or the innocent "Can I grab you for five minutes Meesh before you go?" that could easily happen five times in a row. And, of course, there was no time to look after myself, once I'd tried to make up for lost time with my family.

I know now that I was lacking boundaries, useful approaches and, to some degree, the courage to draw an appropriate line in the sand that distinguished where my supportive role as a leader, employer, co-worker, mentor and even friend began, and where and when it needed to finish. Plus, to reiterate an important point, I often wasn't best placed to provide ongoing support. These days, with better knowledge and my own frameworks for talking about mental health and as both a trained Mental Health First Aid instructor and a Mindfulness-Based Cognitive Therapy instructor, I'm not only better equipped to support people, I'm clear on boundaries and that helps and protects both me and anyone I might be supporting. In fact, by being more boundaried and better equipped, I have greater capacity to help more people.

Are you a fixer? Well, that means you're bound to also be compassionate, kind and caring, but fixing isn't necessarily the way. The good news is I'm here to show you a different way, one that can have better outcomes for all, where, by giving less of yourself, you are able to give so much more.

JOIN THE MOVEMENT

By embracing this book (and I really hope you do!), you are joining the growing movement of people who have the courage to talk about and ask about mental health, a community that is chipping away at the negative narrative, busting myths and booting stigma along the way. Before you've even finished reading it, you'll be feeling like you can either start a conversation with someone to let them know you are struggling with your own mental health or initiate a conversation with someone to find out whether they are perhaps struggling with theirs. But it doesn't stop there – I'm going to do my best to convince you that talking about our mental health isn't only awkward, it can be joyful too!

Warning, there may be tears of joy, sadness and laughter along the way, but as I say to audiences if I'm feeling particularly fragile just before I share my story, I might cry, but please don't worry, I *will* stop (and so will you).

What I hope this book does most of all is convince you that whilst talking about mental health IS AWKWARD, you can absolutely transform that feeling from panic into power, YOUR POWER and the sooner you embrace it, the sooner you and those around you will benefit from it …

Let's get awkward.

CHAPTER 1

My Story, My Why

"I was born with an enormous need for affection, and a terrible need to give it."

Audrey Hepburn

There is nothing particularly special or extraordinary about my story. WAIT! That's not an invitation to stop reading – stay with me! What I mean is that compared to the many people who have experienced any kind of burnout, depression or debilitating anxiety disorder or illness, my story isn't so utterly different or unique; it's not necessarily any more or less painful, dramatic or awful than anyone else's and, look, it's really not a contest. What I've discovered in speaking publicly, privately and, I guess, so openly about my experience of mental illness, is that actually *most* people have a story or experience of poor mental health themselves. Not necessarily their own experience (although I'm still flabbergasted at the sheer number of people who disclose their mental illnesses to me), but what I've noticed is that for a topic that carries so much stigma and secrecy, it's interesting that once you start talking about it, *everyone* seems to have a story or experience relating to mental ill-health, whether it's someone they know or their own. It's everywhere. It affects every one of us in some way.

So, I don't write that my story isn't that out of the ordinary to belittle it, but more to make the point that we *all* have mental health, we are all vulnerable to developing poor mental health and many of us have both first-hand and second-hand experience of it. We've all got a story, it's just that I'm willing to talk about mine, say it out loud, usually including most of the grisly details. Why? Why do I want to share, rake over and now write down, some of my most challenging health issues and experiences again and again? Well, because I truly believe we need to do as much as we can – both collectively and individually – to banish the stigma surrounding mental ill-health as quickly as we can. It will benefit us all. It will save lives.

What I have found extraordinary in sharing my story is that its ordinariness is what people connect and relate to. When I share my story, someone will always share theirs back. So, for as long as it's working, I'll keep on sharing.

REGRETS, I'VE HAD A FEW

"No regrets!" is a popular rallying cry I've often heard myself championing when I share how I feel about my mental illness. But, on reflection, whilst I no longer feel ashamed of my mental ill-health, and in no way do I regret that aspect of my life, I do have some regrets, and it feels important to acknowledge them, for the lessons they offer and the reminders they have become:

- I regret the time given to excessive work rather than spending it with my family and friends and how that impacted on my mental health and wellbeing.
- I regret overriding joy and contentment with "loyalty and responsibility", only to discover that they were both misplaced.
- I regret the occasions (there were many) when I should have stood my ground for what I believed to be the right reasons rather than try to be the peacemaker or avoid conflict, both in and out of work. I regret the impact those times had on my confidence, self-esteem and mental health.
- I regret placing my own health and happiness so far down my priorities that they had fallen off the list, out of sight, out of mind and, in particular, the impact that had on my fertility.

These days, it's about how I frame regret, or perhaps *reframe* it, as we'll explore in Chapter 4. I have regrets, but I do not hold on to them. I cannot change the past, but I can learn from it. I can choose to do things differently now, and in the future, because of those past regrets, whilst not ruminating over them. It's how we deal with regret that is the important outcome of experiencing parts of our lives that didn't feel good and that we wish we had done or dealt with differently, better, or not at all! So, yes, I have

3

regrets – there, I said it. I am also truly filled with a gratitude for life and for living and every single one of the experiences that have shaped me. It's when we hold on to regret, without reframing it or making peace with it, that it gnaws away at us, feeding off us, like a parasite, hidden, yet hurting us, destroying us in some cases and it doesn't have to be that way. We have choice. We can choose to halt our suffering and pain. Talking of pain and suffering …

SO, WHAT ACTUALLY HAPPENED?

Well, 2016 had simply been "One.Of.Those.Years". We all have them. I had led Livity through a multi-million-pound investment deal to grow our business and, importantly, our social impact for young people. The business landscape was volatile and uncertain, the world in general even more so. I had increasingly challenging physical health issues, which were unresolved. One of these was a permanent headache, which I was fondly calling my "investment headache" and putting down to the even longer days I was spending on the investment deal. There was also so much going on at home and the rushing and running felt even greater than usual.

I had some challenges in the business that felt incredibly hard to deal with and, sadly, the fun that had been at the epicentre of Livity's success and growth had all but disappeared for me, something I wasn't even fully conscious of yet. The years of fighting for and proving that you could place equal importance on purpose and profit were taking their toll and the emotional responsibility I felt for not just the team and young people coming through Livity, but for *all* young people everywhere, was weighing me down. I had very few boundaries in my professional life and that was not serving me well. I was neglecting to look after myself and every night for months on end during that year, I would arrive home, having mostly held myself together at work, and find myself unable to stop crying, unable to explain why and usually drinking a bottle of wine to take away the pain (it didn't). The next day I'd put my leadership mask back on and attempt to hold it together until I got back home, and it started all over again.

Promises, Promises

I had promised myself that once the investment deal closed in June, I would head to the doctor's to sort out the headache and buzzing in my ear and that I'd also start going a little more slowly with a greater sense of balance – yes, that's what I needed, more balance. Interestingly I promised nothing to myself in terms of the stress and unhappiness I was feeling; it didn't even occur to me that I might have a choice to do things differently, such was the depth of the wormhole of workaholism I'd fallen into. The deal took longer to close, so I promised myself again, "When we close the deal in July, I'll begin to look after myself better." When we eventually closed the deal in August, the promises to myself and my health went out of the window, as I made the unwise decision to be a "brilliant and dedicated businesswoman" and embrace the theory and importance of "the first 100 days of any new role or relationship"... Oh yes! We'd double down (a ridiculous business buzzword that might as well be code for "work even harder") on getting the new board relationship, and dynamic of having an investor in the business, off to the best of starts! I mean, it wasn't as if we weren't working really hard already, so of course this was nonsense, but this is how I was wired. And so I continued to work really, really hard.

Day 110

Fast forward to 110 days post the close of the deal, at the beginning of December 2016, on the day the removal team were packing up our house. We were moving out for a while to complete some house renovations (just another task on the list of pretty stressful life events). Having just returned from an unusually traumatic business trip to Tunisia, I sat at the bottom of my stairs and thought, "I just can't go on." I was utterly broken; I wasn't sure what was wrong with me, but I knew I needed help. I called my doctor and amazingly got a same-day appointment (an almost impossible feat usually) and I headed there, in a huge personal brain fog. I was clearly very physically unwell by this stage, but there, asking for help, I found I couldn't stop crying. I felt destroyed.

There were a few more doctor's appointments to address the physical challenges and work out a medical plan of action and each time I would sit in front of her and cry and cry and she'd book me back in for another check-up. She encouraged me to take time off from work to address my ill-health, but it was hard for me to get to a place where I felt I could do that.

Talking Heavy Periods Around the Boardroom Table

It was interesting how, at this stage of my ill-health escalating, it was far easier to talk to my board co-workers about my heavy periods, rapidly growing fibroid, severe anaemia and the fact that I was going to have to have a hysterectomy, than it was to talk about my mental health, which I had nervously flagged just prior to the "sitting at the bottom of the stairs, unable to go on" moment. Interesting, because let's face it, talking about heavy periods around the boardroom table, well, we're not quite there yet, are we? But that was by far the easier topic, which just underlines the stigma that talking about mental health still has in even the most open and progressive of businesses. In fact, bringing my physical ailments into the conversation was a welcomed diversion from the slight tumbleweed moment that the tentative words, "I'm a bit worried about my mental health" had sparked a few weeks earlier. I must say, I was entirely complicit in all of this. I felt pretty bad and embarrassed about my list of physical health challenges, but so much more ashamed and a complete failure in terms of how I was feeling mentally and emotionally. This was all in the lead-up to Christmas.

Burnt-out Purpose and Passion

Christmas was a horrible blur. It was a relief to be able to stop and rest and get away from work, and I was still doing a pretty good job of applying the smiley mask of "Merry Christmas everyone, isn't it fun?" but what happened next was just so awful and unexpected. To my horror, I realized that not only was I burnt out physically and mentally, but in the space that I had created to rest and stop, my purpose and passion for the business I had built and loved so much had utterly burnt out as well – the joy had simply gone. A feeling of panic began rising almost at once as I felt sure I wouldn't be able to even walk back into the office we'd built the business in for so many fun and meaningful years, let alone lead it through the next four years of the business plan. This was a devastating moment for me, in what was already an extremely vulnerable state, and that's when the anxiety started escalating rapidly and I entered what felt like a constant state of terror and insomnia.

The Cloud of Shame

It was in the new year, as I prepared to step out of work for a while, that the throwaway remark, "It's a bit awkward when you talk about your mental health Michelle" was made. I was feeling like a time-consuming bore and burden, even when it came to the task of communicating my temporary departure to the wider team. I will never forget the way my cheeks burned as I received those words, stood in the middle of the open-plan office, people all around, getting on with their day-to-day jobs. I stood there feeling so awfully small already as a result of everything that had been happening and then shrank even more as the words landed. My eyes pricked with tears, the hugest lump rose in my throat, my head felt foggier than ever, and my chest felt frighteningly tight, my heart was racing, and my legs were like jelly. I was completely lost for words, my "mask" was slipping, and I needed to escape which I did, but the problem was that cloud of shame shadowed me right the way home.

THE DIRTY DUO

Looking back, I suspect what I call "The Dirty Duo" of depression and anxiety had been lingering within me for some time and were quite comfortably disguised and hidden in the day to day of my life and work for a good part of 2016, and, as it turns out, far longer as I discovered on my journey to recovery. Mental ill-health comes in many different forms. For me, it was quite linear – the burnout happened, then the anxiety kicked in and escalated at a startling rate and then the depression, already sitting at a deep level, rose like the hugest of waves ... and not in a joyful "surfs up" kind of way. I'm a terrible and fearful swimmer, so to be engulfed by the sea and a huge wave is literally a living nightmare, and that was how it felt. Worse still, I began flip-flopping between the two states, making what I was experiencing even more confusing.

Looking back now with my Mental Health First Aid instructor hat on, there were many signs throughout 2016 (oh, yes, and you know, throughout my whole life before that moment, as I went on to discover) but gosh, The Dirty Duo really let loose once I had stopped working. Alternating between the two states of depression and anxiety was exhausting and terrifying. For me, in short, anxiety was characterized by feeling *everything*, whilst depression was feeling *nothing*.

My "That's Me" Moment

When I stepped out of the business, I continued to feel unable to talk about the true depth of the problems I was experiencing – neither was I able to explicitly ask for and accept help and support. That remark, alongside my own self-stigma, really had struck so hard and deep. I knew that I needed to do something to help myself, something secret, a private way of taking care of myself that meant I didn't have to leave the house, my bedroom, or even at times, my pyjamas. I downloaded the

Calm App, co-founded by the brilliant and inspiring Michael Acton Smith, who I now refer to as one of my burnout buddies, having shared the stage with him to tell our burnout and entrepreneurial stories. I didn't personally know Michael at this time, though, I was just desperate to find some way of quietening my increasingly chattering and noisy mind. I also bought and was slowly reading Ruby Wax's book, *A Mindfulness Guide for the Frazzled*.

I was at the height of a paranoia and insomnia I had never experienced before, the ear-shattering noise of wakefulness in the silence of the night made my heart pound as my thoughts became more and more irrational, yet so terrifyingly real. I was carrying huge shame and guilt about not being at work, I was feeling like a burden to my husband, Remi, and a complete and utter failure in all areas of my life. In the moments I could muster the energy, I would force myself to do something to address the "pathetic" state I was in. I would listen to, or more like just play and not hear a word of, a daily Calm meditation or follow some mindfulness from the book. It's funny how we can be listening, yet not hear a single word, isn't it? I then reached the chapter where Ruby movingly describes falling into an episode of depression whilst writing her book. Here it is ...

Depressed ... no end in sight. I suppose this is my brain saying, "You went too far, you pushed me too far, and now I'm shutting down for the season. I'm going to shut you down, make sure you can't do anything even if you try." In a way, it's survival; when your thoughts have declared war on you and you feel friendless, hated and forgotten, the brain just shuts down, leaving a hazy blur, a fog. I've been in the fog for about a week. It feels like I've been reunited with an evil lost relative, someone from my past I can vaguely recognize – and then it comes to me: oh yes, it's depression. I remember now. When you're well, you can't remember you ever had it. Probably your mind ingeniously erases it from your memory because it's too frightening for you to contemplate it ever coming back. And now that my depression is back in town I have that "aha" moment that this is what it is. This feeling of being estranged from my body and mind is depression. Of course.

Oh my God, does my heart go out to people with depression who have to go to work and feel what I'm feeling! To have to drag the heavy weight and then try to hide it in case people think you're wallowing in some phantom sickness. The horror that, if someone asked you to tell them what the matter was, you couldn't. No one is as cruel to those of us who have depression as ourselves. We keep ourselves going even when we are broken. It's like beating a dying animal to keep it moving. I'm amazed that so many people keep on going to work and trying to act as if everything's okay. They should be knighted or given something like a Purple Heart for their bravery, because that is the most difficult thing on earth when you're depressed: to have to keep acting like a human when you don't feel like one anymore.

... I'm fortunate that I can just sit this out, because I don't have a nine-to-five job. I can just lie here. I'm babysitting myself: waiting, waiting, for the gigantic thing that has blocked out the sun to move away.

From *A Mindfulness Guide for the Frazzled* by Ruby Wax, published by Penguin Life.

With tears rolling down my cheeks as I read her words, I shouted silently to myself, "THAT'S ME! What she's describing is how I am feeling, but hang on a minute, she's calling it depression." I felt each word, sentence and paragraph had been written solely for me to read. It was what I now call a "That's Me" moment and it was what got me back to my doctor and into a very honest conversation about how I was *really* feeling and, critically, accepting and moving into treatment for a diagnosis of clinical depression and anxiety.

The combination of reading Ruby's experience and getting a diagnosis was a game-changing moment. Until then, I just hadn't had the words, the language, or maybe even the permission and courage to describe how I was really feeling. Within her description, not only did I read what I was feeling, which created a sense of connection and helped me feel less alone, I also read and felt hope in her words and that book. I'll be forever grateful to Ruby for sharing her story so honestly and openly. This is the first of many examples beyond my own that demonstrates the impact and importance of talking about our experiences of mental illness. Sharing stories creates connection, helps us feel less lonely, nudges us gently toward support, and then to heal and pass it on. By sharing our own challenges, we help others toward support more quickly.

The Dirty Duo have been a part of my life for a very long time; it's just taken an equally long time to work that out. The episodes of depression and anxiety (and to an extent the burnout) I've experienced handfuls of times before were maybe not to the extremes of that particular time in 2016, which was akin to an 8.2 on the Richter scale, but looking back it feels like they've been a background tremor in my life for a long time, just never formally diagnosed.

Let's Create More "That's Me" Moments

A big part of my personal mission is to create more "That's Me" moments for others. And once you experience one, or have one pointed out to you in a book, you notice they happen all the time, even more so when you Own *Your* Awkward and help others own *theirs*. They can give us the courage to ask for help, and they help us connect and have empathy and understanding; they are a sign that we are both listening and hearing, all so crucial for offering help that is truly useful. They are as much about the good as they are about the bad and the ugly, and they can be wonderful chain reactions and examples of paying it forward and smashing stigma, one brave story at a time.

That's NOT Me Moments

It's worth noting, we won't connect with everyone's story and experience, we are all different, we're all unique with a personal story and experience that begins from before we are even born. Our individual stories are what shape our resilience, our vulnerability, the factors and happenings that we have or haven't experienced that have made our lives more difficult or challenging and, on the flip side, more protected or joyful. No, we won't connect with everyone's story, but to play our part in making it easier for us all to talk about our feelings and how we are coping, neither should we judge, simply because we don't understand. We must seek to understand, connect and, if we can't, we should just work on the non-judgement bit.

LOSING MYSELF IN ART

When listening to the Calm App (let alone actually doing the mindfulness) or reading Ruby's book felt too hard and overwhelming, and believe me it often did, I would simply stare into one of the pieces of artwork we are lucky to own. Artists have a wonderful way of swapping art if they are both admirers of one another's work, and so because of my husband Remi's own art career and his network of artist friends and contemporaries, we have some beautiful pictures and paintings.

We had moved out of our home whilst renovations took place and were holed up in a sweet ground floor flat, belonging to our good friends, only five minutes away from home in the car, but a different postcode and an area we'd not spent much time in previously. I've found this beneficial in helping me to visually compartmentalize one of the most difficult times in my life, away from my actual home.

Whilst we only had the bare bones of our belongings with us, Remi had taken great care to make sure we had beautiful walls and artwork around us, to create a sense of home, if only temporarily, and so, in my more difficult days and hours, I spent a lot of time losing myself in different pictures, in particular an artwork by our friend and artist Jaybo Monk. I would look at his painting and see so many different things – an angel flying, a woman falling, sky, sea, waves, clouds as well as joy, pain and very occasionally hope. I felt like I was in the picture; I felt like I *was* the picture. It was like Jaybo had climbed inside my head, sat and quietly watched for a while and then climbed back out and painted what he'd seen onto canvas. I would stare at the picture as a way to calm my chattering and unkind mind; at other times I'd stare deeply into it trying doggedly to ignite some kind of life and feeling into the lonely, hollow pit of my mind. Sometimes it worked. How curious these two such different states could be tended to by one picture. Our art pieces became both my sedatives and stimulants, depending on how I was feeling and what I needed. The powerful role that art can play to help and heal the mind stayed with me and was to become an important part of my "What Next" in life.

AT THE DOCTOR'S

With tears rolling down my cheeks yet again, I tentatively explained to my doctor how closely I had related to Ruby's description of depression. I remember feeling such a sense of relief as I said it out loud and my doctor responded so calmly, with such kindness, and then got straight into the practical. I'm pretty sure that had I been able to see the invisible thought bubble over her head it would have said "No shit Sherlock" as I confided to her what I was experiencing and feeling. A discussion about medication versus talking therapies followed and she gave me some reading materials on SSRIs, a type of medication that treats depression. We agreed she would refer me for some phone-based therapy and I would come back the following week to see how things were going and make a decision about taking medication.

FIRST STEPS

I urge you to talk to your doctor if you are struggling with your mental health. It's the best first stop if you're not sure where to start. I am grateful for the care and consideration my doctor gave me – not everyone will always have such a positive experience (but many will!). If you don't get the response you deserve and are hoping for, ask to see another doctor and don't give up until you find someone you connect with, who you feel is able to help you. Repeat, don't give up. Of course, I understand this can be easier said than done, especially if you are struggling with your mental health, but this book can help you with this, so please, stay with me. One step you can take is to consider asking a friend or family member who you trust and can rely on to go to the first appointment with you.

Being Offered Meds

I read the blurb describing the SSRIs for depression and, to be honest, I felt pretty fearful about trying them. My hesitancy was partly because my doctor had explained that I'd need to commit to them for at least six months and that felt uncomfortably close to the looming hysterectomy. But it was also because I was still feeling immense shame and failure about the state I was in, and for me medication represented a next level that I wasn't ready to admit nor embrace. Whilst being given a diagnosis of depression had been somewhat of a relief, taking medication all seemed a bit serious, a bit scary and I had too many "what ifs", which I should have discussed with my doctor, but didn't. Clearly I wasn't Owning My Awkward at that stage, I was just consumed by it.

Of course, now I understand what hogwash and how unhelpful and self-stigmatizing that kind of thinking and labelling is and, heck, maybe I'd have made a speedier recovery had I embraced the meds, but at that moment I felt like I just wanted to try the talking option first. Despite feeling stuck in the lowest of lows, there were fleeting moments when I could sense that there *might* be a light at the end of this long tunnel, despite not even seeing or feeling even a flicker or glimpse of it just yet, but there had to be surely? However, the less fleeting, more permanent, thoughts and feelings would unhelpfully rage away, leaving me exhausted and feeling less able than ever to make a decision about the medication. I think in the end I just put the leaflet into one of my admin boxes, out of sight, out of mind (quite literally!) Luckily, the therapy phone appointment landed and at least there was now something to focus on. A date.

FIND YOUR THERAPY, FIND YOUR THERAPIST

The first course of talking therapies wasn't a great experience for me, but importantly it *was* the first step. I had a couple of calls and whilst trying not to be too dismissive of the experience, I pretty much immediately dismissed and ended the sessions. The early stages of getting help can be deeply confusing and hard. Patience and perseverance were two of the first lessons I had to learn.

Just as I was feeling I'd taken two steps back and a little lost once more, a woman called Christine Neillands came into my life through a recommendation from a friend and co-worker. Christine practises hypnotherapy as well as several other talking and listening therapies. Her slightly alternative approach to the talking therapy the doctor had referred me to felt safe, nurturing, non-judgemental and incredibly supportive. I immediately felt she understood my pain and utter burnout with such empathy (a skill and quality we'll go on to explore) and we began weekly sessions.

Around this time, on one of the days I could summon up the energy to get out, I went for coffee with my friend Geoff McDonald, an ex-Vice President of HR at the global firm, Unilever, and Co-founder of Minds@work. Geoff was in the early days of publicly sharing his story of mental illness, from the other side of the dark tunnel, in the light of recovery. As I described to him how I was feeling, he shared that he'd experienced something similar. He described it as anxiety-fuelled depression and said there was someone he thought I should speak to who might help. And so, from another "That's Me" moment of connection,

Geoff introduced me to Dr Annemarie O'Connor, Chief Growth Officer of a psychological therapy practice and platform called HelloSelf, who in turn introduced me to Dr Rumina Taylor, who became and still is my psychologist.

Feeling Seen and Heard

This proved to be an incredibly helpful combination for me. Rumina uses Cognitive Behavioural Therapy (CBT) techniques, which I found really useful for dealing with challenges in the present and moving myself forward, and Christine was particularly brilliant at helping me recover from and let go of what had gone before. I cried during most of the early sessions with both Rumina and Christine as the pain and trials and tribulations of the last year or so poured out of me. What still strikes me is how supportive and non-judgemental they both were; they both did a fantastic job of helping me feel less alone and less pathetic about how I was feeling. They acknowledged my pain, and that made a real difference to me. When they started to help me normalize my feelings, make sense of them and feel less ashamed of what I'd been thinking and feeling, things began to really shift. They both gave me a strong sense that given what I was sharing with them, it was no surprise that I'd hit a wall and was struggling with depression, anxiety and some trauma. REPEAT, they weren't surprised, they believed my pain. I can't tell you how much it helped to be seen, to be heard, to be believed.

As well as the combination of talking therapies, I was also getting my physical health into better shape as I hurtled toward the date of my operation. My paranoid feelings were lessening and I was finding ways to manage my chattering mind; the lows still felt low, but not quite so dark and smothering.

MICHELLE, STAY WITH US

On 6 April I checked in to the London Bridge Hospital for my hysterectomy. I was fortunate to have a health insurance policy that covered the treatment. I was now physically recovered enough to proceed with the operation and whilst The Dirty Duo were still very much inhabiting my body and mind, things were feeling less extreme, less awful, less frightening and I was certainly beginning to feel calmer and more stable, if not much "better".

A hysterectomy is a major operation, but straightforward. I was taken into surgery late afternoon and was back in my room just a couple or so hours later. My consultant came to check all was well and then headed off for the weekend. Remi and Lili visited. I was clicking away on the pain relief button, and not exactly coherent I suspect, but so happy to see them both, if a little delirious and sleepy. They too headed home to let me sleep and recover. What happened over the next couple of hours is as hazy in some parts of my mind as it is crystal clear in others ... my blood pressure began to drop. The team, all so lovely, tried to keep me up to date and whilst I was most definitely in a post-op fog, I was beginning to pick up that something wasn't right.

More medical staff arrived and then suddenly I was being taken to a room nearer to the nurses' station so that they could keep a closer eye on me. As I was wheeled into the new room,

I was met with the most stunning view of the River Thames and London Bridge. "The things we do for an upgrade and a room with a view," I piped up, trying to stay jolly and keep the mood light, maybe for myself, but I think more so for the team around me. I remember thinking they were all so warm and attentive in their various roles, so skilled and impressive – there was a real sense of working as a team, something I greatly missed. The number of people in the room increased and out of nowhere I was receiving a blood transfusion and hazily signing an alarming waiver document as I needed to go back into surgery. I could feel the vibe and tone of the team and room had shifted. I heard the words that I'd been trying not to ask come out of my mouth, "Am I going to be okay?" Just as my legs started bouncing up and down uncontrollably, someone said, "Stay with us, Michelle." Someone else followed up with, "Hold on, Michelle." I remember thinking, "Oh wow. That's what they say on TV when things are getting really dicey" and then "Does this mean death? You are kidding, this? Now?" and then, "I do not want to die, I want to hold on." I felt so calm, clear and alive, and then it all went dark.

Stepping into the Light

Spoiler alert ... I lived! That amazing team saved my life. I came around in the Intensive Care Unit, a day or so later, and then it was back up to my room with a view. I remember being awake in the middle of the night and Dean, the ward night manager – my angel who had stayed with me at every stage of the emergency – coming in. He told me how amazing I'd been throughout the ordeal. At that moment, with the most beautiful light of the moon glistening on the River Thames and shining into the room, it did all feel pretty amazing. I felt pretty amazing. I was so incredibly grateful to be alive.

Recovery

My recovery from the operation was slow and painful, and my mental recovery also took a knockback. The seriousness of the haemorrhage and what I had experienced stayed with me and I found myself replaying the situation over and over in my mind. I felt sad as well as incredibly shocked. I also had a huge amount of gratitude for surviving and recovering.

I think the shock was amplified in response to the timings of the last six months and I couldn't help wondering whether, had my operation and the haemorrhage that followed happened earlier in the year, at the height of my depression, I might have lacked the energy, or may have even decided not to "hold on" or "stay". I found that a frightening and deeply sad thought, because it made me realize just how awful I had felt for so long.

It is often said that people who take their lives by suicide do not do so because they want to die, but because they cannot live with the pain they are experiencing. Of course, who really knows whether my resolve to "hold on" or not really made any difference to my survival, but the clarity of that moment, making such a conscious decision to hold on, stayed with me and still does. The experiences of the past few months percolated like a pot of 1980s' coffee and a sense of clarity emerged. I was so completely grateful for being alive and despite the ups and downs in my life, I knew I wanted to keep living and to do that fully, freely and healthily. I needed to make a huge shift. I needed to come completely out of leading the day to day of Livity and I wanted to give this little idea I'd been gently playing with a chance to develop to see if it and I could make a difference in the world. I had a new purpose emerging and it felt scary, but good.

THE PJS I COULDN'T GET OUT OF

During all this time of burnout, anxiety and depression – and then hysterectomy and haemorrhage recovery – I spent a heck of a lot of time in my pyjamas, often because I couldn't face getting out of them, sometimes because I was simply going slow and recuperating. As part of my own treatment for the depression and anxiety I'd given myself permission to play with the work question, "If I did it all over again, what would I do? No brainer, I'd start another purpose-led business" (she thought from the depths of the burnout and depression that the first business had caused). But what? Isn't the work mantra "Do what you love?" Uh oh. I'd hit a brick wall immediately, as I still had depression, wasn't passionate about anything, and I didn't love myself, never mind anything else.

I stayed stuck in this cycle for some time until one day I must have reached the crossroads where brilliance meets madness (to be fair, the place where all great ideas come from right?), and the PJs that represented everything holding me back became my inspiration. Did other people ever see the duality of the "PJ day", both good and not so good? The good PJ days when we joyfully choose to stay in our jammies all day – resting, recuperating, watching box sets, reading the paper, eating delicious food and simply just "being". But then for some of us, there are the days when we can't get out of our PJs or out of the front door; we might not even be able to get out from under our duvet covers. These days are depression, burnout, anxiety and more; these days are poor mental health.

I wondered if we could make the most kind and caring pyjamas, designed by brilliant artists (remember how art had been so key to my recovery?) and use the PJs, their packaging, the platform from which we sell them and the people we put around them, as a way to share stories of hope and help. Could they be a way to make mental health an everyday conversation and banish this notion that talking about our mental health is in anyway awkward? Could I take the words, "It's a bit awkward when you talk about your mental health" that had been so crushing, silencing and stigmatizing and make something positive out of such a negative and awful time? And could we call them Pjoys (see what I did there)? In all honesty I wondered if maybe I had lost my mind. I said the idea out loud to my husband Remi, who didn't laugh and said he would love to design a pair. I shared it shyly with my best friend Susie, who also didn't laugh and said that she thought Pjoys was a brilliant idea. She loved the purpose and said she would love to help me get it off the ground as a way of creating a positive legacy for her dear brother and my friend, Dave, who had taken his own life just a few years before.

Pjoys – PJs With Purpose

Pjoys – PJs with Purpose – was born on 8 March 2019, International Women's Day, after smashing our crowdfunding campaign launched on World Mental Health Day in October 2018. Gently tapping into my entrepreneurial and creative skills, Pjoys helped me organize my continued recovery around a renewed purpose – making mental health an everyday conversation. We've sold many pairs of pyjamas, raised money for and shone a spotlight on the good work of numerous mental health organizations and charities and, most importantly, we've started thousands of conversations about mental health.

TRY THIS …

I've shared "my why", now it's your turn. Take a moment to reflect on why you are here, why you are curious about getting comfortable with uncomfortable conversations and why you want to own your awkward.

Why do you want conversations about mental health to be easier? Why is it important to you?

You might want to write it down, you might like to say it out loud or just simply let it bubble away in the back of your mind. If you're not sure, it's okay, keep reading, it will come.

THE CORNERSTONES OF AWKWARD CONVERSATIONS

Confidence

Taking very small, private steps, with no pressure attached, helped build my confidence to start talking about how I was feeling.

Capability

Just getting going, talking and starting the conversation was the important first step for me. Sometimes you've just got to start. Getting better at and more comfortable with conversations grew from there.

Communication

Seeking out and connecting with other people's stories gave me helpful language to describe how I was feeling.

Compassion

Finding and working with therapists who I connected with meant I felt seen and heard, which helped me move more comfortably into receiving help from them.

CHAPTER 2

What is Mental Health Anyway?

"You cannot hope to build a better world without improving the individuals. To that end, each of us must work for his own improvement, and at the same time share a general responsibility for all humanity, our particular duty being to aid those to whom we think we can be most useful."

Marie Curie

Confidence: a feeling or belief that you can do well or succeed at something; in our case, that's a conversation about mental health. Speaking of which, what the heck is mental health anyway? If we're here to build our confidence to talk about it, we'd better make sure we understand what it is. And so, in this chapter, as well as providing some explanations and definitions that will help give you the fundamentals and foundations of what mental health is and the global challenge it presents, I'm going to share with you why language matters and how it can fuel stigma, how our mental health moves (hold onto your seats folks), how we are all so very unique and how when we understand that of each other and ourselves we are better placed to step into the space of non-judgement, a crucial aspect of successful conversations. We're also going to reference suicide, and why it's important to talk about it up front, regularly, awkwardly maybe, but critically. We're not going to hide it at the back of the book because we are too nervous to talk about it. With all of the aspects of this chapter, please take care of yourself and seek support if it brings anything up for you.

In Mental Health First Aid England training, we describe mental health as being about:

- How we feel, think and behave
- How we cope with the ups and downs of everyday life
- How we feel about ourselves and our life
- How we see ourselves and our future
- How we deal with negative things that happen in our life
- Our self-esteem and confidence
- How stress affects us

For a more theoretical view, I also like the World Health Organization's definition of mental health outlined below. It presents the higher starting place of "health" and that our physical *and* mental health are part of our overall health and, importantly, that the two are inextricably linked and can impact one another both positively and negatively. Note the use of the words "vital concern".

"Health is a state of complete physical, mental and social wellbeing and not merely the absence of disease or infirmity. Mental health is a state of wellbeing in which an individual realizes his, her or their own abilities, can cope with the normal stresses of life, can work productively and is able to make a contribution to his, her or their community.

"Mental health is fundamental to our collective and individual ability as humans to think, emote, interact with each other, earn a living and enjoy life. On this basis, the promotion, protection and restoration of mental health can be regarded as a vital concern of individuals, communities and societies throughout the world."

And so, with all that in mind, do you know what? We *all* have mental health.

THE MENTAL HEALTH CONTINUUM

Let me bring that to life. The first thing to acknowledge is that we all sit on and move around the Mental Health Continuum (created by the American psychologist Corey LM Keyes). I've found this Continuum to be one of the most effective tools, both in and out of MHFA training, for helping people understand that our mental health is not fixed and that problems escalate if we don't get help. If we accept that we are all on this Continuum – that we all have mental health – we can begin to develop a greater sense of understanding and empathy for both ourselves and those around us.

The Continuum is a super-useful tool to plot or check in with your own mental health, where it is now or even has been in the past. Once you are familiar with the Continuum, you can use it, with care (remembering it's not your job to diagnose), to support a conversation with someone else about their mental health.

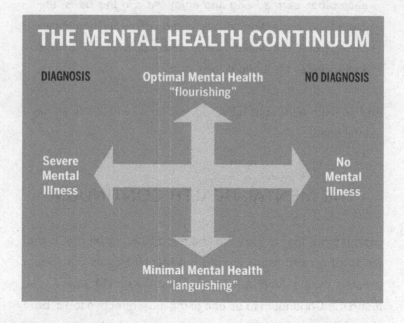

The horizontal axis plots how we might be described in terms of the medical state of our mental health, including whether or not we have a diagnosis of mental illness. The vertical axis plots our wellbeing, our wellness, our mental fitness. When we're at the very top of the vertical axis, we're mentally fit and have optimal wellbeing – we might even be described as flourishing. If we're at the bottom, we're missing that sense of good wellbeing and mental fitness. Sometimes we might even find ourselves stuck there, languishing. Let's look at each of the four quadrants.

Moving Around the Four Quadrants

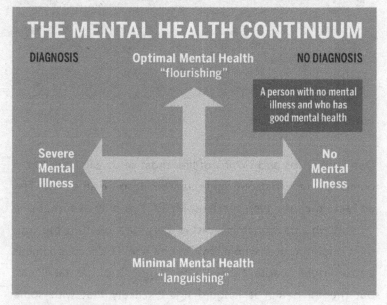

THE MENTAL HEALTH CONTINUUM

DIAGNOSIS

Optimal Mental Health
"flourishing"

NO DIAGNOSIS

A person with no mental illness and who has good mental health

Severe Mental Illness

No Mental Illness

Minimal Mental Health
"languishing"

Top-right quadrant

The top-right quadrant represents a person with no mental illness or disorder who has positive mental health and wellbeing. The majority of us start here, come back here and probably tend to hang out in this quadrant the most.

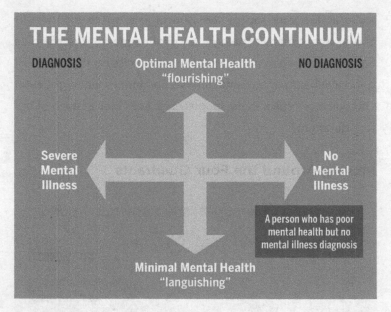

THE MENTAL HEALTH CONTINUUM

DIAGNOSIS   Optimal Mental Health   NO DIAGNOSIS
"flourishing"

Severe Mental Illness

No Mental Illness

A person who has poor mental health but no mental illness diagnosis

Minimal Mental Health "languishing"

Bottom-right quadrant

Due to the ups and downs of life, most of us will have found ourselves in this bottom-right quadrant at some time in our life. (In fact, in all my time teaching MHFA I've only ever met one person who passionately insisted they had been in the top-right quadrant their whole life. One person. Lucky chap.) In this bottom-right quadrant there is no diagnosis of mental illness, but mental health is languishing. It's likely that with some support, a shift in self-care or even simply time, we'll move back up to the top-right quadrant pretty quickly, reflecting the ups and downs of life. The problem arises when we find ourselves stuck in this quadrant, perhaps not talking about how we're feeling, hiding it, covering it up even and not moving back up to the top-right quadrant. Because you see, when we talk to a mental health professional about how we're feeling, we can begin to get help and support to move us back up to the top-right quadrant or, in some cases, we'll receive a diagnosis of a mental illness, at which point we move across to the bottom-left quadrant. The point is we keep moving and that is a good thing.

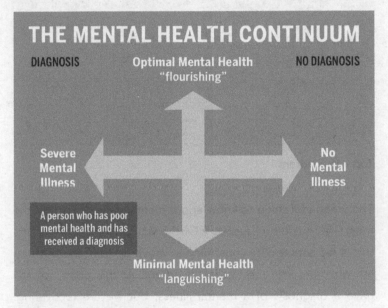

THE MENTAL HEALTH CONTINUUM

DIAGNOSIS   Optimal Mental Health   NO DIAGNOSIS
"flourishing"

Severe Mental Illness   No Mental Illness

A person who has poor mental health and has received a diagnosis

Minimal Mental Health "languishing"

Bottom-left quadrant

In this bottom-left quadrant there is a diagnosis of mental illness. We're not necessarily feeling any better – in some cases we may experience even greater issues, but we have acted. We've asked for help and, with support, we can now receive treatment. Again, we keep moving and this is a good thing.

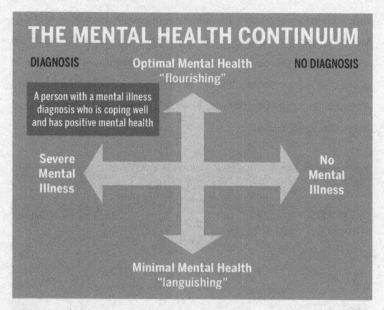

THE MENTAL HEALTH CONTINUUM

DIAGNOSIS   Optimal Mental Health   NO DIAGNOSIS
"flourishing"

A person with a mental illness diagnosis who is coping well and has positive mental health

Severe Mental Illness

No Mental Illness

Minimal Mental Health
"languishing"

Top-left quadrant

The wonderful thing to know about mental ill-health is that the most likely outcome is recovery. On the Mental Health Continuum, this is represented by continuing to move up from the bottom-left quadrant into the top-left quadrant. At this point, we still have a diagnosis of a mental illness, but we are recovering. We have a greater sense of contentment, an ability to cope, more confidence and a brighter and more hopeful outlook, and therefore our wellbeing has improved. We're experiencing fewer symptoms of our mental illness. We're feeling better. We keep moving – this is a great thing!

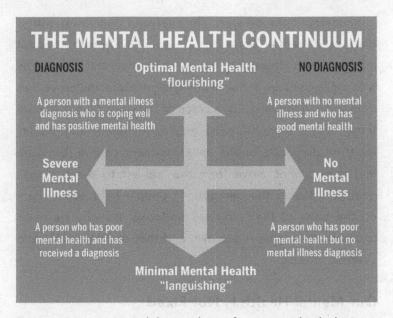

THE MENTAL HEALTH CONTINUUM

DIAGNOSIS

Optimal Mental Health
"flourishing"

NO DIAGNOSIS

A person with a mental illness diagnosis who is coping well and has positive mental health

A person with no mental illness and who has good mental health

Severe Mental Illness

No Mental Illness

A person who has poor mental health and has received a diagnosis

A person who has poor mental health but no mental illness diagnosis

Minimal Mental Health
"languishing"

Recovery: moving round the quadrants from top-right clockwise to top-left

Some people move all the way around the quadrant, back to the top right, with a sense of "full recovery". Others may have received a diagnosis that they live with for a longer period of time or maybe even forever. This doesn't mean they remain constantly unwell or that they won't experience good mental health and wellbeing. It is possible to flourish with a good sense of wellness, with a diagnosis, in the top-left quadrant and it can be as equally positive as the top-right. Of course, from either the top-left and top-right quadrants we can move down and round again, either with the same or a similar mental health issue, or a different one. We keep moving – this is life.

Recovery looks different for everyone and living with a diagnosed mental illness doesn't equal living with constant mental health issues. It's important to know this, as people with a diagnosis are at risk of being stigmatized and prevented from moving forward into a place of recovery. Plus, there are those with a diagnosis who may no longer strictly qualify for their diagnosis based on assessment criteria, but who feel they cannot move from the top-left to the top-right quadrant due to the perceptions people hold about them on the basis of their original diagnosis. It's why we need to eradicate stigma – our own and that of others. Oh, and keep on moving.

Our Mental Health Is Not Fixed

I've witnessed the Mental Health Continuum help people identify that they've been or currently are stuck in the bottom-right quadrant. When they've been able to say it out loud, it's been such a gift to offer an ear for them to talk about how they're feeling and encourage them toward seeking professional help. For me, it's a conversation starter and a self-care tool and it can be for you too.

And you know what? We'll keep on moving up and down and round and round the Continuum. The point is to watch out for either ourselves or others being stuck in either one of the bottom quadrants or even the top-left if we no longer fit the diagnosis. Our mental health is not fixed, and we should never feel stuck. There is always help. There is always hope.

SULKERS

It took me until my mid-40s to really begin to understand better the many aspects of myself, including my mental health. There were clues of course, even in my childhood, when I would be described as sensitive at best, moody or sulky at worst. I remember what felt like a massive inability to express myself and there often being confusing feelings of deep hurt accompanied by sudden low self-esteem in response to things that happened or things that were said. For some people these might feel like minor, everyday challenges that they would be quick to recover from, but they seemed to impact me in a starker more emotional way and often for longer.

In my 30s, I had one of those "That's Me" moments whilst listening to a radio programme on "sulkers". There was an insight that sulking might be the suppression of a verbal reply because of the fear of saying something so awful that might cause irreparable damage to a relationship, such was the person's hurt or anger. It was massively comforting to know that I wasn't alone or the only one to think and feel in such a way.

Then there was the moment in my early 20s being gripped by what I am now able to identify as most likely a panic attack whilst walking to work. My job was stressful and pressurized, at a time when my self-care was at a low, fuelled by what I might once have described as partying, but what I can look back upon as using alcohol and drugs beyond what might be described as recreational, and more to dampen, mask or artificially change my feelings. On that occasion I went to my doctor as soon as it happened, as I was really frightened. I was signed off sick and prescribed medication. I remember the doctor saying, "I'll give you this particular type of medication, as it's prescribed for issues that don't need to show up as anxiety in your notes. You don't want this on your medical record." Fuelled with shame, I barely left my flat for a number of weeks and was then "let go" from my job. Just what I needed. I didn't take the medication, and I don't think I really needed to in that instance – time and talking to friends helped, once I felt brave enough to. I eventually got back on my feet and into a job that felt more purposeful.

STIGMA AND MENTAL HEALTH

As we've seen, it's the stigma of poor mental health that often prevents or stops people moving around the Mental Health Continuum. So, what is stigma? This is how I see it:

- Stigma is negative, stigma is fear; it's lacking in knowledge, empathy and truth.
- Stigma is unkind, it's judgemental; it's in our words, our body language and also our culture.
- Stigma drives conscious and unconscious bias, and in turn that drives discrimination.
- Stigma stops people asking for help or moving forward.
- Stigma is not clever or helpful and it's not funny.
- Stigma is a shard in the heart of awkward.
- Stigma kills.

You, here, in this book, embracing The Cornerstones of Awkward Conversations are playing your part in identifying stigma, extracting it from the heart of awkward and giving it the boot. As we'll continue to find out, awkward is okay, stigma most definitely is not.

MY LITTLE SISTER AND THE "BIG C"

Susie Shaw is the Founder of the charity, Mind Over Cancer. She is a trained counsellor, and a Mental Health First Aid instructor. She is also my wonderful sister. For two decades she played an important part in changing the cancer narrative in the UK by targeting and empowering young people to take ownership of the awkward, scary and stigmatized topic of cancer and change the story and conversation. She shares a hopeful insight in that the subject and stigma of "mental health" is where cancer was 25 years ago. We all knew that we should talk about cancer, but we didn't know how to and so we didn't, because there was such stigma and fear attached to the topic. We even referred to it, in hushed voices, as the "Big C", not wanting to say it out loud in fear of people's reactions and driven by our assumption that there was no recovery from it. But information is power, and after years of education, we now talk about cancer on a daily basis and about the importance of early diagnosis for better and quicker recovery outcomes, all of which are the same messages with mental health issues.

> And here's the great part, it's all within us. Susie says:
> *To get people talking more easily about cancer we didn't have to go out and train everyone up to be nurses, we had to simply create a safe environment to start the conversation and smash the stigma.*

Words Matter

The power of our words and the language we use or don't use, can't be emphasized enough. A misplaced word, an unthoughtful description or a throwaway comment all fan the flames of embarrassment, fear and ultimately stigma and, as we're learning, stigma stops support, stigma stops recovery and, tragically, stigma sometimes kills.

Think about how we might misuse language in subtly stigmatizing ways. For example, we might say "I'm so depressed", when we mean, "I'm feeling fed up" or "You are so OCD" to describe someone's preference for tidiness and order. Depression and OCD (Obsessive Compulsive Disorder) are both diagnosable mental illnesses that can be debilitating for the person experiencing them. To incorrectly use the diagnosis and definition undermines the reality and pain of people who are truly experiencing either one or another mental illness and may hinder, or worse, prevent them seeking help.

And, finally, it's not only the words and language we use to describe others, but also those we use for ourselves. Self-talk, self-labelling and the narrative we create for ourselves is often unkind, harsh and lacking in compassion. Maybe that gives us a clue to where we can start to create change?

TRY THIS …

Bring to mind as many words and phrases as you can that feel negative, unhelpful and judgemental ways of describing poor mental health in others. Try not to overthink it, just go for it. Write them on a pad or in a journal, note them on your phone or laptop, or even say them out loud, knowing this is a safe space for uncomfortable conversations if we remain open to learning.

So, take a deep breath and give me the best of your worst! I want your "Crazy", "Insane", "Nutters", as well as the more subtle, yet equally unhelpful, "mentally unstable" and "disturbed". Just sit with those words for a moment. How do you feel? How do they make you feel? What do they make you think? Comfortable? Uncomfortable? Write down how you feel if that helps.

Now bring to mind words and language that feel more neutral, non-judgemental and positive ways to talk about other people's poor mental health. Here we are looking for accurate and appropriate descriptions like, "experiencing depression", "a person who self-harms" or "living with general anxiety disorder" or even more neutral phrases like "they are accessing support" or "they are experiencing a mental health problem". Similarly, stay here in this space for a moment. What do you notice about the two different parts of the exercise?

We do a similar version of this exercise in MHFA training, and it always plays out the same way, as it most likely has done for you. It's far easier to do the first part of the exercise than the second ... and, oh wow, you can feel the awkwardness in the air as we set it up. The negative, stigmatizing words come thick and fast onto the paper, whilst the positive and non-judgemental words and terms languish; a few words and phrases are slowly added, but it feels much harder to do, with far greater discussion and debate.

It's always interesting to me how people pretty much immediately get the point of the exercise. We more readily use unhelpful, stigmatizing language in our day-to-day lives – it's true, isn't it? It's years of stigma at work, plus the influence of both the media and entertainment industry and how mental health is or isn't portrayed.

"YOU'RE SO CONTRARY, MEG"

Meg Mathews is an icon. Described as "The First Lady of Britpop" in the 1990s, she was the third most written about woman during that time, after Princess Diana and The Spice Girls. These days she is a menopause campaigner and the author of *The New Hot*. I met Meg at a conference and, after formal introductions, we fell into an easy conversation filled with connection – about mental health of course! Sitting on the floor whilst we waited our turn to share our stories with the audience, Meg fed me CBD Gummy Bears, which, to her relief and joy, is about as "rock 'n roll" as it gets these days. Meg went on to take part in our official Pjoys launch at Fenwick on World Mental Health Day. She told me:

Mum was a worrier... that's what we called it when I was growing up. I think I was also always a bit of a worrier as well. Anxiety certainly escalated for me during the 90s when I was under the spotlight all the time. It would grip me suddenly. I'd get ready to go out, but then be struck by such anxiety that I'd have to pull out of the commitment, whether it be interviews, dinners, parties or opening nights, every time feeling awful about letting people down. My anxiety would rise even more as I worried that I was gaining a reputation as unreliable and somehow difficult or "better" than others. One day a close friend described me as "contrary". It really hurt, it felt like they didn't know me or understand what I was going through at all. And then I hit 50 and the menopause. My anxiety went through the roof and I felt overwhelmed all the time. I didn't understand what was going on. There were other symptoms, but I didn't have the language or knowledge to be able to talk about it. Luckily someone else did and once I understood that I was perimenopausal, I realized

I could do something about it (after I'd got over the shock!). I've also been diagnosed with ADHD and Dyslexia as well as Post-Traumatic Stress Disorder from the impact of the media intrusion. The pursuit of perfection was so prevalent back then, it made it almost impossible, and of course awkward, to tell people when you were struggling. Even me, as someone who has always been very open. Therapy, knowledge, changing the language and learning to "not sweat" things going wrong, has not only helped, but it's also been so freeing. That "contrary" comment no longer has any hold over me and I'm happier now than I've ever been.

It helps to think about your words before you say them out loud and be aware that what might seem like a throwaway comment can mean so much more to the person on the receiving end of it. "You are so 'contrary' Meg." and "It's a bit awkward when you talk about your mental health Michelle." Words that (sometimes) make our cheeks sting even years later.

STIGMA? LET'S TALK ABOUT SUICIDE

Due to the stigma of suicide, asking someone if they are having suicidal thoughts might be the most awkward conversation of all. So, what better reason to learn how to Own Your Awkward and be the person who has the confidence to act, to ask, to talk about suicide so that other people feel like they can too.

A note of caution: While talking about suicide is a good thing, if it brings up difficult feelings for you, please look after yourself whilst reading this section. Talk to someone you trust if you feel affected by any of the information or stories.

Let's continue to understand the enormity of the issue of suicide through some statistics:

- One person dies by suicide every 40 seconds around the world, according to the World Health Organization.
- Suicide is one of the leading causes of death in young people worldwide.
- UK research found that 1 in 4 people will experience some kind of suicidal thinking in our lifetime and you are more likely to encounter someone experiencing suicidal thoughts than you are someone having a heart attack … another reason to place equal importance on MHFA training as well as physical first aid.

One of the most important confidence-building messages about suicide, which I'm always keen to share, is that you won't make someone more likely to act upon suicidal thoughts by asking them if they are experiencing them. The understandable concern that we might make a situation much worse, or put thoughts and ideas into someone's head, often stops us from starting a conversation that is simply coming from a place of care and concern. It means we may halt a conversation before we've even started for fear of saying the wrong thing. What if, though, by asking someone if they are experiencing suicidal thoughts, you are opening a door that will help them talk about their feelings and what if that makes the biggest difference to them? Evidence shows asking someone if they are suicidal can protect them, give them permission to talk about and validate their feelings, and people who have felt suicidal have described the relief from being able to talk about what they were experiencing.

GOING QUIET

Susie Moore is a Global Brand Consultant and my partner in Pjoys. We have been the best of friends since our early teenage years. I so wish I had been a Mental Health First Aider when she needed it the most. Here she shares her brother Dave's story and how she could relate some of it to mine, and then her part and purpose in bringing Pjoys to life.

Meesh went quiet in 2016 and I didn't know why – no responses to emails or calls. In 2017 I knew why – I found out what she had been going through, and that she was coming through it.

My brother Dave went quiet in September 2010, but for good. He didn't manage to get through his depression, and he took his own life. He was the life and soul of a party, loved by everyone, and a best friend despite being a younger brother! But on the inside he was struggling; we just didn't know how much until it was too late. We know now. He expressed himself in the letters, beautiful poetry, photographs, music and playlists he left us. But somehow it was too "awkward" for him to express himself in conversation, and so we missed the opportunity to help him. I believe if he had been able to talk about how he was really feeling, we could have helped him, and maybe he'd be here today. So when Meesh was recovering from her depression and told me her idea for using PJs and art as a way to help make mental health an everyday conversation "because no one should ever feel awkward talking about their mental health", I couldn't not get involved. Dave wrote in his letter, "Don't let my life be in vain, there was too much good in it", and this was the opportunity I needed to do that, and to create Dave's legacy.

We said right from the start that Pjoys would be worthwhile if we could save one person's life, and this thought has inspired us with every activity or event that we do. From the feedback we get we know we have started hundreds, perhaps thousands, of conversations and made a small but significant difference to many people's lives. Simply through sharing stories and, very joyfully, using PJs and art as the conversation starters.

Not being able to find or say the words to share how you are feeling. Not being able to find the strength to share how you are feeling. Not wanting to burden others. Embarrassment, shame, weakness, self-loathing, awkwardness and stigma. These are the things that stop people from talking about suicidal thoughts they might be experiencing, and this is where The Cornerstones of Awkward Conversations and my BRAVE and SENSE frameworks can help.

MY LIFE FOOTPRINT VERSUS YOURS

As we're learning, stigma and judgement often get in the way of communicating about mental health and make things more "awkward". When someone's life and experiences are quite different to our own, it may be more difficult to understand their challenges and difficulties, which can create judgement, and well, greater levels of awkwardness, right? One way of tackling this is to have a greater understanding of your own and other people's "Frame of Reference", a term first coined by the psychologists Jacqui and Aaron Schiff to attribute to the individual filter each of us has on reality.

Your Frame of Reference is how you make sense of the world, other people and yourself. We each have our own Frame of Reference that feeds into our beliefs, feelings and behaviours and is influenced by and evolves through every interaction, event and circumstance that make us, well, us.

- It's about where we were born, how we were born, our family situation and size, our early childhood.
- It's about our education, hobbies and interests, our aspirations, likes, dislikes and the cultural influences that surround us.
- It's about gender, relationships, genetics, personality, sexuality.
- It's about our achievements, the things that have shaped us and our lives and, of course, it's about the ups and downs of life and how we cope and recover.

All these elements, and more, influence and shape how we see the world and therefore how we understand, view, experience and respond to life, day in day out, good times, bad times, joyful times and yes, also those painful times. Visually, I like to think of the Frame of Reference as our "Life Footprint" – like our fingerprints, our footprints are unique to us all, walking through life, sometimes skipping, always carrying the weight of us and shaping our story, step by step.

TRY THIS ...

Get your preferred writing utensil if you love a list and want to immerse yourself in this exercise, or at the very least do a version of it in your head. This exercise will help you step back and consider how you see the world, and how that might form and maybe sometimes communicate bias, judgement and stigma or equally, and hopefully more often, what shapes your compassion, empathy and ability to connect with others.

The question is, what is *your* Frame of Reference? Your Life Footprint? Each prompt will help you paint a picture of what makes you, you. Your Frame of Reference affects every interaction and communication you have and how you respond to and support people with emotional and mental health issues, demonstrating once again, how understanding yourself can do wonders for supporting others. This is the groundwork for using the SENSE and BRAVE frameworks (see Chapters 5 and 7) and as we get into them, you'll discover how understanding and working with your own Frame of Reference can help you have more confident and compassionate conversations.

Consider the following:

- Place of birth
- Early childhood
- Age
- Gender
- Sexuality
- Race
- Ethnicity
- Socio-economic background
- Hobbies and interests
- Education
- Likes and dislikes
- Aspirations
- Disability
- Chronic illness
- Family situation
- Relationships
- Work
- Mental health
- Physical health
- Spirituality
- Achievements
- Values
- Cultural influences

This exercise is a great way to take stock of your life and what has shaped it and you – you'll find the good and the bad (and most definitely the ugly, so brace yourself), as well as the joy and the pain. If doing this exercise brings up any difficult feelings for you, stop, take a break and consider talking to someone about how you're feeling.

DISABLED PEOPLE AND MENTAL HEALTH

My friend Sulaiman Khan is the Founder and Chief Purpose Officer of ThisAbility Limited. He told me:

My experience is that disabled people are rarely included in the wider mental health conversations and our mental health needs are not taken care of. For example, every time I see a specialist for my physical disability, they never check on my mental health. The only time it's mentioned is when I have my yearly care package review and they ask, "Are you suicidal?" There needs to be a lot more support and a more holistic approach that includes disabled people and our wisdom and richness in this space.

I'm Pretty Resilient Actually

Whilst the key part of the story I'm sharing in this book is about my experience of mental ill-health, I'd actually describe myself as a pretty resilient and strong person in many ways, especially when I look at my own Frame of Reference. Co-founding Livity in 2001 was a leap, a risk and an experiment, as well as being incredibly exciting with a great big vision for solving and plugging what was missing in business, in our communities and, to be honest, in the world as we saw it.

I left a secure job and bunch of co-workers I loved, said goodbye to my fun convertible MG, and lost all sight of security – this was huge for me, as many of my fears and anxieties revolve around financial security and independence, shaped undoubtedly by my home life in my teenage years. It's worth noting that those same fears are also my drivers and motivators, which now, with stronger and clearer boundaries and perspective around them, are helpful. Financial moments of jeopardy for Livity were frequent, not only in the start-up years, but also as we grew, and sometimes as we shrank. My house and good credit rating often came to the rescue, always with a belief that it was the right thing to do, for our purpose (young people), for our Livity people (wages and jobs) and for the rent and running costs (business responsibility), but it always came with an accompanying weight of terror, as the house providing insurance against loans and overdrafts for the business was putting a roof over the heads of myself, Remi and our daughter Lili. Providing the security personally always came with a feeling of sickness in the pit of my stomach and a chattering head full of "what ifs". That said, it was often matched with an absolute faith in the business and mine and my business partner, Sam's ability to lead us through and out of the more difficult times, and a strength and resilience that would underpin those moments, both in and out of my work life. Like life, our mental health is not always simple.

Connection

Sometimes we'll find ourselves facing someone whose Frame of Reference and Life Footprint is similar to ours, sometimes a little different and at other times perhaps a galaxy or two away.

When you notice any negative thoughts and judgements arising in response to what someone is sharing with you, bring to mind the Frame of Reference, or the image of your Life Footprint, using it to remind yourself that we are all different and that what is mentally difficult and painful for one person might be a ride in the park for another. Use it to help you step into a more non-judgemental, empathic headspace and ensure difference doesn't get in the way of a good conversation or, worse, stop one from even starting.

By being aware of our own Frame of Reference and curious and compassionate about someone else's, we can use it to tap into both ours and theirs, to find connection and kindness, which will help everyone Own Their Awkward and keep that conversation going and glowing. And remember, as the author Maya Angelou, wrote: "We are more alike, my friends, than we are unalike."

WHY WE NEED TO OWN OUR AWKWARD

Let's look at the global rationale, the human need and the business case for taking the deep breath to Own Our Awkward and ask for or offer help. To effectively strengthen our Confidence, Capability, Communication and Compassion, we've got to understand the bigger context and, trust me, it's really big. When we consider the startling number of people across the globe who are struggling with their mental health on a daily basis and the impact that has on them, those around them and the world at large, it's clear that Owning Our Awkward, silencing the stigma and addressing the multitude of issues that arise as a result of avoiding a conversation about mental health is not a "nice to do"; it's essential.

I want to expand your compassion and awareness for just how many people are affected, often hidden in secrecy, by mental ill-health. Your improved confidence and compassion will support and grow your sense of capability and communication as we get into our talking frameworks SENSE (see Chapter 5) and BRAVE (see Chapter 7).

A Global Crisis

We are experiencing a global crisis in the space of mental health:

- The World Health Organization has deemed "burnout" a recognized workplace phenomenon.
- Depression is the leading cause of disability worldwide.
- In November 2020, the global cost of mental illness to the world economy was estimated at US$2.5 trillion according

to *The Lancet*, the UK's leading and globally renowned medical publication, and projected to increase to US$6 trillion by 2030.

Mental health is a global priority. We live in a world where 1 in 10 people live with mental illness. Mental health problems and mental illnesses have substantial economic costs for individuals, communities and nations. These costs can be incurred directly, arising from the use of health and other services, or indirectly from lost work, social and educational opportunities, the effects of stigma and discrimination, and reduced life expectancy.

More than 800,000 people die by suicide every year. Suicide sits among the top 20 leading causes of death globally, number 15 more specifically, just below HIV/AIDS and just above malaria. If that wasn't tragic enough, for every adult who dies by suicide, it's estimated that more than 20 others have attempted suicide. Death by homicide, conflict and terrorism sit on this morbid line-up of leading causes of death, at numbers 17, 29 and 31, respectively, showing that greater numbers of people are killing themselves rather than one another.

The Hidden Costs

More than an estimated 12 billion days of productivity are lost worldwide because of the effects of depressive disorders and anxiety disorders alone, at a cost of US$1.15 trillion. Presenteeism is reduced productivity whilst at work due to mental ill-health that is not being supported properly (or maybe at all). It is those times that many of us can relate to when we go into work despite the fact we are not well. The cost of depressive disorders relating to presenteeism is estimated to be 5–10 times higher than the cost of depression-related *absenteeism;* those times when we are officially off work due to mental ill-health, demonstrating once again how fear, stigma and a lack of understanding and awareness drives the notion that mental health issues are not deemed as serious as physical health issues, making them more difficult to take time away from our jobs to address and recover from. Of course, presenteeism statistics are more difficult to measure and there is a sense they are underestimated, because presenteeism is often about hiding our mental ill-health; it's about showing up, whilst not truly showing up, it's the mask we apply on the way to work and keep on throughout our working day and often beyond, because we can't talk about it, because it's uncomfortable, difficult, risky, vulnerable ... because it's awkward.

Research from 2017 estimates that a total of 970 million people, i.e. 13% of the global population, have a mental or substance use disorder. Here's what the breakdown looks like by different disorders and types of illness:

- 264 million – Depressive disorders
- 284 million – Anxiety disorders
- 46 million – Bipolar disorder
- 20 million – Schizophrenia
- 107 million – Alcohol use disorder
- 71 million – Drug use disorder
- 16 million – Eating disorders

Although worldwide figures give us some idea of the scale of the problem, it's important to recognize that these figures are estimates and are affected by different factors. Mental illness is widely under-reported in many countries and all these difficult global stats and stories are experienced from places that might be described as more privileged or underprivileged, which also skews the numbers and the deeper understanding of the impact of mental illness for many.

Whilst we've already acknowledged mental ill-health is not a competition, an individual's vulnerability to developing poor mental health is something we should be aware of. There will be those who are vulnerable to mental ill-health and are most likely already tackling challenges that the majority of us will never experience, for example:

- In countries where there is conflict, famine, poverty or dictatorships.
- In communities that may be the target of bias, whether conscious or unconscious, stigma, bullying and exclusion – black people and people of colour, disabled people, those affected by abuse, people who are neurodivergent, and lesbian, gay, bi, trans, queer, questioning and ace (LGBTQ+) people.
- For those experiencing unemployment, trauma, uncertainty, and many more.

As we saw in the Frame of Reference exercise on page 49, we all have a unique life story and set of circumstances that play their part in influencing whether there is an increased likelihood of us experiencing mental health issues.

CORONAVIRUS

A 2020 paper in *The Lancet* highlighted the urgent need to tackle the harmful impacts of the Covid-19 pandemic on mental health. The paper warned that the pandemic could have a "profound" and "pervasive impact" on global mental health now and in the future, whilst a 2020 survey and report from The International Committee of the Red Cross found that Covid-19 was affecting the mental health of one in two people, and in the UK the Centre for Mental Health released research approximately seven months into the pandemic that estimated 10 million people in the UK (there are 66.65 million in total) would be seeking support for their mental health as a direct result of the pandemic, with 1.5 million of them being children. And it's no surprise. A pandemic presents a direct threat to our lives and the lives of our loved ones and at the time of publishing this book, we're about two years into it. Uncertainty, volatility, isolation, confusion, security, loss, ongoing uneasiness, change, and more, for all of us in so many different ways began to impact all areas of our health almost immediately in early 2020. We're now beginning to see and feel the longer-term impact on our mental health and we need to be able to talk about it now more than ever. Because our "mental health" was in crisis before Covid-19, it almost feels like a ready-made pandemic to follow the pandemic.

THE CORNERSTONES OF AWKWARD CONVERSATIONS

Confidence

Now you better understand the mental health context and issue.

Capability

The Mental Health Continuum is a great tool for demonstrating how we *all* have mental health and that it is not fixed.

Communication

We've learned how the power of language can be both helpful and unhelpful.

Compassion

The Frame of Reference helps develop more compassion by providing you with the clues to understand what makes you, you and reminders that we are all different. And don't forget, whilst it can be difficult, it is a good and compassionate act to talk about suicide. It may open the door and help someone talk about what they are feeling. It could save a life.

CHAPTER 3

Why We Feel Awkward

"How very little can be done under the spirit of fear."

Florence Nightingale

Let's step back into that moment when either I'm going to tell you about my mental health or ask you about yours. I don't know how it's going to land, what your response is going to be or what either you or I will say next. Worse still, what if what follows next is SILENCE? A really, LOUD AWKWARD SILENCE?! Or, what if you laugh at me or I laugh at you? What if you start crying or I do? In these moments, whether we are asking someone how their mental health is, telling someone how ours is or, indeed, if we are on the receiving end of somebody telling or asking us, the truth is, we might be feeling vulnerable, fearful and naturally trying to protect ourselves from any negative reactions or emotional bullets and grenades that may head toward us in response to our words. So what's happening to trigger all these feelings and how can we more easily recognize and manage awkward, rather than IT managing US?

FIGHT, FLIGHT OR FREEZE

In those moments of fear and panic, we've most likely and unknowingly triggered our Fight, Flight or Freeze response, the survival instinct that stems from the days of cave women and men, when our body and mind would work together to give us a shot of adrenaline and cortisol hormones (and more) to either fight, run or hide from the bear. These days the perceived threat may occasionally be as dangerous as the bear (heck it might still be the bear in some places far beyond London!), but as the world has evolved, stress levels have risen and mental health issues are made up of all kinds of contributing factors. Some of those factors trigger that natural survival instinct in a way that is disproportionate to the actual danger and threat, but nonetheless challenging for many of us. The panic element of fear is even less helpful as it prevents reasonable thought and action and is often contagious – panic breeds panic. None of which is useful when offering help or asking for it. It's at this point perspective can be useful, especially if it's the thought of having an awkward conversation that's igniting this response.

Is It Really Fear?

Gavin de Becker is widely regarded as the USA's leading expert on the protection of public figures and is the Chairman of Gavin de Becker Associates (GDBA). His work in the prediction and prevention of violence has earned him three presidential appointments and Oprah Winfrey describes him as "the US's leading expert on violent behaviour". As if the endorsement from Oprah wasn't enough, the actor Meryl Streep described his book, *The Gift of Fear*, as "A thorough and compassionate primer for people concerned about their safety and the safety of their families." Frankly, I'm sold.

He says, "Real fear occurs in the presence of danger and will always easily link to pain or death." The book's core purpose is to teach us how we can best use our fear response to alert ourselves to *real* danger and threat and how when we find ourselves in an almost constant state of what *feels* like fear, but where there is no real danger or threat, it can directly impact and diminish fear's true power and effectiveness for keeping us safe and being able to respond to danger. That doesn't sound good, does it?

Gavin introduces two rules about fear that he believes can improve your use of it and reduce its frequency:

- "The very fact that you fear something, and its possible 'dreaded outcome' is solid evidence that it is not happening, because fear summons our predictive resources, serving to tell us what *might* happen next, not what *is* happening now."
- "Know that *what* you fear, is rarely what you *think* you fear – it is what you *link* to fear, i.e, harm, death, pain, rejection. In truth, most fear happens in just two places; our memory and our imagination."

Circle all of that back to the fear of having awkward conversations and the case for avoiding having them is fading. Why? Because although our Fight, Flight, Freeze response is triggered, it's not really fear but a *sense* of fear that unrealistically, unhelpfully and unnecessarily holds us back and stops us from helping others, and indeed ourselves, which is a tragic and missed opportunity. As Gavin says, "True fear is a survival signal that sounds ONLY in the presence of danger. Yet unwarranted fear has assumed a power over us that it holds over no other creature on earth. If one feels fear of all people and situations all of the time, there is no signal reserved for the times it is really needed."

Worry and What Ifs?

"In my experience, it's the awkward conversations that almost always turn out to be the best conversations," Katharine Woodcock, headmistress of Sydenham High School in London shared with me. "With the challenges and barriers to starting what feels like an awkward conversation mostly stemming from 'worry and what ifs?'" The question is, are worries and what ifs really worth the time and energy? If you're getting the gist of things, then I think you're not going to be surprised to learn the answer ...

Worry, wariness, anxiety and concern all have a purpose, but they are not fear. So anytime your "dreaded outcome" cannot be reasonably linked to pain or death and isn't a signal in the presence of danger then it really shouldn't be confused with fear. Gavin de Becker describes worry as a fear we manufacture – that it is not authentic. He offers the insight that worrying about something is a choice that is often providing us with a secondary reward or excuse. Here are some examples of the whats and whys you could find yourself worrying about that might prevent a conversation from even starting:

- To avoid change or admitting powerlessness over something – *I won't mention their mental health because, really, what can I do?*
- To protect our connection to others, to show love – *I won't mention their mental health in case I make them feel worse.*
- To protect ourselves from disappointment or hurt in the future – *I won't tell anyone how I'm feeling in case they don't understand/care/want to help.*

The thing is worry will not bring solutions. It will more likely distract you from finding solutions. Conclusion? Worry is not fact. Worry is not real fear. Worry is a waste of time and energy. And so, my friend, worry not.

THE SOCIAL ASPECT OF THE BRAIN

As well as the Fight, Flight, Freeze response being stimulated in such a physical and primal way, there's something else that is quite possibly happening for us in those awkward moments and it's all to do with belonging and connection.

From the instant we are born, our brain is trained to obsess with social connections, to obsess with being loved and feeling we belong, because that's what keeps us alive. Our brain has evolved to give us social and emotional skills, rational thinking, the ability to think about the past and the future and to solve problems – and our brain is really really big in comparison to that of other mammals, which, by the way, is why we have to be born ridiculously "prematurely". If we were born when our brains were fully developed, we would be born at the age of two (impossible, but also ouch at even the thought!). As such, in order to survive, before our brains are fully developed and because we are unable to fend for ourselves, we need other human beings to protect us.

As we grow and develop and can begin to fend for ourselves, it's no longer a life-or-death situation necessarily, but the brain still *feels* as if it is. And that's why we care about whether people love us, whether we feel accepted, whether we're part of a group or not, because to our brain social safety equals survival in the first couple of years of life. And those feelings stick.

Thinking back to the awkward pause, or even the potential of the awkward conversation, maybe we are feeling risk-averse to asking someone about their mental health, or telling someone about ours, in order to protect ourselves from any chance of being rejected, pushed away or shunned if our words land in the "wrong" way and cause upset and hurt. If belonging is so important to our primal survival, it's no wonder we're keen to avoid making ourselves vulnerable to being rebuffed or, worse, abandoned. Simply put, we dislike rejection, ridicule and embarrassment, we care about what others think about us, and we will do more to avoid pain than we will do to seek pleasure – could it be all of these evolutionary characteristics that potentially stop us from talking about mental health?

Stage Fright

Gavin de Becker recognizes the importance of belonging and he says surveys have shown that ranking very close to the fear of death is the fear of public speaking and, in turn, the potential loss of identity that attaches to performing badly – all firmly rooted in our survival needs. For all social animals, from ants to antelopes, identity is our pass to inclusion, and inclusion and belonging, as we've learned already, are the keys to survival. Historically, the loss of identity as a member of the tribe or village, community or culture, would have a likely outcome of banishment or death (harsh!). So, the fear of public speaking is not just the fear of embarrassment, it is linked to the fear of being perceived as incompetent, which links to the fear of losing your job, home, family and ability to contribute to the community. The same thinking might fairly be applied to the idea of having a conversation about mental health. The many possible consequences of a conversation that *might* not go well and that *might* result in damage to, or the loss of, a relationship, can prevent a conversation from happening at all. Once we identify and understand the deep-rooted fear response we are experiencing, where it comes from and why, we can hit it with a reality check that, if we let it, will discredit those thoughts and fears.

Make It Personal Michelle

So, about stage fright … Back in 2017, just eight weeks after my hysterectomy and that dicey death moment, probably far too soon to be up and out and about in London, let alone France, I was stood in the wings of one of the main stages at the Cannes Lions International Festival of Creativity, about to step onto the stage and present to about a thousand attendees. Mark St Andrew, the then Head of Communications for the festival, had invited me to speak. His brief was "Come along and just tell your story. Make it personal. Be really honest, and just trust me that there will be people there who want to hear it. Oh, and it should be a talk that nobody else should be able to give."

What's the saying? Go hard or go home! Well, there was no way I was going home. I stepped onto the stage, under the glare and heat of the lights, wearing a pair of spray-painted pyjamas and a headset mic that made me feel like Madonna (sadly, without the voice), and began to tell my story of burnout. I can't pretend that I didn't feel massively awkward for most of my time on stage, and it was not the most amazing and joyful experience of my life in the moment. It was all going on: the sweaty (me) silence and anticipation (the audience), red cheeks, dry mouth, pounding heart and a million "What ifs" (all me). I took a deep breath and looked into the audience to make some eye contact and human connection. I couldn't see a single face due to the glare of the lights shining back at me. Taking another deep breath, I simply looked on and into the brightness and began to share my story.

How did it go? Well, it's all a bit of a blur for me and you know, it was okay, probably better than okay, but it's kind of hard to toot your own horn sometimes, so here's Mark tooting it for me: "Sometimes you find a speaker that gets it. Someone who understands the power of a story well told and how it can inspire others – often in surprising ways. Michelle is absolutely one of those people. Mixing personal experiences with practical advice and her serene stage presence, she totally killed it. It was a thrill to see a room full of people respond the way they did and Michelle was the speaker everyone wanted to meet. Her authentic, witty, unpretentious and quietly inspirational style is as powerful as it is calm."

Aww shucks and no mention of it all being a bit awkward then? You know, it was a shared risk and I'm not sure how much of a powerful storytelling plan I had in advance. I just felt deeply that there was a massive unspoken secret in the Creative and Media Industries and way beyond, affecting so many people who were feeling awkward and embarrassed talking about their mental health.

"It's a bit awkward when you talk about your mental health Michelle" was beginning to become my power and not someone else's weapon. It was the response from so many different people that I received after the session that gave me the greatest sense that sharing such a personal story was a good, perhaps valuable act. Who would have thought that getting my PJs on, standing up tall and talking honestly about my burnout and mental health challenges would be the start of something so meaningful for me? The start of my amazing "What next?" in life.

THE ELEPHANT IN THE ROOM

Jonny Benjamin MBE is an award-winning mental health campaigner and the Founder of Beyond – a youth mental health charity. He is also the author of *The Book of Hope*, a book of personal stories that will create ripples of "That's Me" moments for many of its readers (and that I proudly contributed to). His 2014 social media campaign with Rethink Mental Illness to #FindMike, the man who talked him out of jumping off a bridge when he was suicidal (and

who turned out to be a lovely chap called Neil Laybourn, not Mike at all), went viral and led to Jonny becoming a prominent spokesperson on the subject of suicide. I knew Jonny would get the idea of awkward and bring inspiration to it. He did and despite, or perhaps because of, the challenges he has experienced, here he is bringing laughter and smiles to his awkward:

I've had LOTS of awkward conversations surrounding my mental health. I'm also gay and from a Jewish community so there's been a huge number of awkward conversations around that too. The most awkward conversations I've ever had took place after I was diagnosed with Schizoaffective Disorder and put into a psychiatric hospital at the age of 20. When I was finally discharged, my mental health became the "elephant in the room" among my family and friends. Looking back, it makes me shudder to think just how enormous this "elephant" actually was. At every occasion we got together, we tried to avoid the subject at all costs. Thankfully, at the age of 34, I can now safely say that discussions about my mental health (and sexuality) have become so much easier to have. This is partly due to the reduction of stigma in our society, although I think we still have a long way to go until we achieve "parity" between mental and physical health, but I'm hopeful we will get there. Learning to laugh about it has been a blessing. I'm often a very serious person. I always have been since I was a kid. But I do have a lighter side too.

> *Applying this lightness and finding the humour within the awkwardness has taken time and practice but I realize now the value of it. Taking a step back from the situation, getting in touch with your breath and body, and smiling at your awkwardness is a start to Owning Your Awkward. It might feel strange and unfamiliar at first, but with practice it gets easier, like everything in life.*

GIVING AND GIFTING FOR SURVIVAL

As we're discovering, humans are social creatures and motivated by bonding and connection, and there's more to back this up and help us understand what shapes our behaviours and reactions. There's evidence of gifting and its benefits throughout all human history – it helps us maintain social bonds and is a way of showing gratitude for the contribution that another person has made to our success and wellbeing; it also sets us up for times in the future when we might need support from others. Giving gifts is a way to contribute to our long-term safety and success in our community – and, here we are, back to the importance of belonging.

As well as evolutionary survival, of course, there's also a simple reason to give someone a gift and that is it makes us feel good and others feel good. It's a positive feeling. Gifting brings us joy. Giving someone your time, attention, care and love by talking and listening might be the greatest gift of all.

Giving Away PJs

When the Covid-19 pandemic hit in 2020, it would have been easy to launch a loud commercial Pjoys campaign encouraging people to buy our PJs as WFH (Work From Home) became our norm and rallying cry. To be honest, we needed as much of a commercial boost as possible to keep going and growing and so it was tempting to go all out on WFH! But it didn't feel right. There was so much uncertainty, fear and tragedy raging, we felt something different was needed.

I drew inspiration from a book written by J Kelly Hoey called *Build Your Dream Network (BYDN)*, which I'd bought in 2017, just at the point when I was beginning to see and feel some sense of recovery and future for myself, as I waded through the treacle of depression and anxiety. Knowing I needed to explore a different professional path, but totally unable to see what it looked like, my starting point, inspired by Kelly's book, was to simply meet with and talk to people in my circles and networks. It was exhausting and daunting in what was still such a vulnerable state, but I had a lot of cups of tea and the odd glass of wine with loads of lovely people and the human connection was good for me. Kelly shares the idea of "Give Give Get" when building connections and ultimately a strong network – when you give more than you ask for, you get more back. I loved the idea, in both her context and beyond, and to this day do my best to live by it.

During the pandemic we applied "Give Give Get" to our Pjoys activity. We donated sample fabric we were storing in the UK to a local sewing group, who turned it into 100 pairs of scrubs. We bought and donated PJs found languishing in the same factory our PJs were made in to a charity called Solace, which provides refuge for women and children escaping violence and abuse. We put on free "Bedinars", online conversations about mental health, and hosted free mindfulness sessions. We saved unused fabric, again found in our factory, from being landfilled and used it to make a more affordable range of PJs called Revive. We created the Reloved Robes range, made by our friend and seamstress Annie2Pins in Peckham, from pre-loved sarees, sourced from Gayatri, a female entrepreneur in India. All these activities felt good and because of them we were able to start even more conversations about mental health.

THEY OWN THEIR AWKWARD (SO THAT YOU CAN OWN YOURS)

Yes, awkward is uncomfortable and most of us will know it and experience it. If we open our eyes though, we have examples all around us of people who go about their lives Owning Their Awkward brilliantly, from goths to geeks, EMOs to entrepreneurs and trainspotters to comedians and, of course, that friend, co-worker or family member we all have and love. There are plenty of people who already embrace awkward as a key part of who and what they are, and we can learn so much from them.

Monsters and Gremlins

Steve Chapman is an artist and writer, beautifully immersed in his work of exploring creativity and the human condition. He is also the king of owning his awkward and celebrating it. In fact, I'd almost describe him as making a career out of his awkward these days. Honestly, he is the most joyful example of a human embracing his wonkiness and encouraging others to do so with theirs. He is a big inspiration, and he came into my life about an hour or so before I stepped onto the stage in Cannes. Steve's talk was just before mine and was about imposter syndrome and the monsters and gremlins in our heads that give us the most unhelpful narratives (and which, by the way, pretty much *all* of us experience at some point in our lives – really, it's not just you). It might be said that they are the same monsters and gremlins that activate the awkward in us. Steve is a brilliant speaker and so the comparison kids were in full bullying force as I stood watching him and waiting for my turn on stage, fuelling my awkward even more and 100% on topic, feeling like an utter imposter. But you know what? I walked onto that stage sweating, yes, but Owning My Awkward and I'm so glad I did.

Viral Awkward

When I chatted to Steve about awkward conversations, one of the many interesting things we talked about was how when someone else experiences awkward, but perhaps doesn't have the awareness, the courage or the skills to own it and activate it in a positive way, it mutates into what we agreed was best coined as "viral awkward", passed on toxically to others, and we know how fast and easily those viruses can spread, don't we?

Steve shared an example from when he worked in the corporate world and was asked to talk to a co-worker, who was described as a "stress case". Steve was asked to "deal with her" because he was "good at the mental stuff". All Steve could hear at that moment were the negative labels and language being applied to the woman and it made him unduly nervous and most definitely awkward. He suddenly felt unqualified to have a conversation with her. His reflection was that the co-worker asking him to do this had passed on their awkward to him, and in doing so the labels and judgement already placed on the person who needed help had rendered Steve awkward too. What, he wondered, would have happened if his co-worker had simply asked him to have a chat with the person because they were concerned about them?

LAUGHTER

The perfect antidote to viral awkward, laughter really can be the best medicine. Jarred Christmas, a New Zealander, is one of the funniest comedians living in his adopted country, the UK. In a moment of seriousness I asked him for his insights on talking about mental health and Owning Your Awkward ...

Push on through the awkward because on the other side there are only positives. As a stand-up comedian, I have found a way to turn my awkward moments into jokes and comedy. To me, this shows that awkwardness and embarrassing moments are a shared experience. We all go through it. Even Tom Cruise has farted at the wrong moment.

TRANSFORMING PANIC INTO YOUR POWER

What is awkward?

- Awkward is uncomfortable
- Awkward is embarrassing and cringy
- Awkward is unwieldy and unco-ordinated
- Awkward is nerves
- Awkward is imposter syndrome
- Awkward is stigma, prejudice, bias and judgement
- Awkward is difficult, tricky and hostile
- Awkward is inconvenient
- Awkward is clumsy
- Awkward is feelings of panic
- Awkward is threat
- Awkward is fear

No wonder on first look we don't much feel like owning it, eh?

Imagine if we used all those awkward feelings to our advantage? Imagine those awkward nerves becoming the indicators that we care. Or that the embarrassment we are feeling being the sign that we are alert, alive and in touch with both our own and other people's feelings? What if we could view uncomfortable thoughts and sensations as merely the messages that we are about to start an important conversation? And imagine if the cringy, clumsy inconvenience of it all could be transformed into confidence and a sense of capability led by compassion? Could reframing and looking at it differently hold the key to us Owning Our Awkward and turning the panic we're feeling into our power?

Let's look at awkward as assets not obstacles:

- Awkward is vulnerability
- Awkward is caring
- Awkward is tender
- Awkward is thoughtful
- Awkward is honest, real and alive
- Awkward is brave and courageous
- Awkward is action and asking
- Awkward is sensitive
- Awkward is power
- Awkward is authenticity
- Awkward is kind

Much better, right?

When we view awkward as an asset, something that is valuable and helpful, it starts to become something we'd be way more interested in, open to exploring and maybe even owning, doesn't it? In fact, being celebrated or admired for Owning Our Awkward could easily be something we'd even like to be described as ourselves, yes?

Wait! Is awkward becoming attractive?

By now I hope that you're beginning to feel much warmer toward this thing we call "awkward" and that you're seeing the benefits emerging. Not only have we explored and understood better the more granular aspects of what awkward is and why we feel awkward when we're about to talk mental health, we're also building a rather beautiful case for why looking at awkward in the opposite way to the "norm" is motivating, exciting and perhaps not as intimidating as we initially thought. Awkward really can be thoughtful, caring and kind.

It's good to do uncomfortable things, difficult things, awkward things. It builds our resilience, flexes new muscles, makes us stronger and, the more we do it, the more we get out of it. We grow, we learn and we potentially give and help more.

Awkward is an Invitation

Talking about mental health is a generous offer and invitation to yourself and to others. The more we embrace it, the more we get out of it and the more we get out of it, the more we have to give to others (Give Give Get!).

It's getting harder and harder to find reasons not to Own Our Awkward, isn't it?

So, how do we do it?

THE CORNERSTONES OF
AWKWARD CONVERSATIONS

Confidence

Remember that *what* you fear is rarely what you *think* you fear – it is what you *link* to fear, i.e. harm, death, pain, rejection. In truth, most fear only happens in two places: our memory and our imagination. Don't let it hold you back.

Capability

Think opposite. Flip those unhelpful definitions of awkward and transform them into assets.

Communication

Look out for the signals and indicators that alert you to your "awkward". Reframe them and activate them for good … so that you can Own Your Awkward rather than it own you.

Compassion

Give Give Get … when you give more than you ask for, you get more back.

FOUR STEPS TO
OWNING YOUR AWKWARD

CHAPTER 4

How to Own Your Awkward

"Power is not given to you. You have to take it."

Beyoncé

We've learned that fear and awkwardness sometimes make us want to instinctively run away and sometimes they see us frozen to the spot. We now know that these are natural reactions and rather than view them as frustrating and awful feelings, we can view them as indicators and signals that can help us create more thoughtful responses and wiser actions. They are what can help us transform "awful and awkward" into "awkward and awesome".

Enter my Four Steps To Owning Your Awkward, a way to communicate with yourself, bolster your sense of capability, guide you into the space of confidence and flood yourself with compassion ALL BEFORE YOU'VE EVEN STARTED A CONVERSATION!

FOUR STEPS TO OWNING YOUR AWKWARD

When you notice the awkward emerging …
1. Stop and Notice
2. Acknowledge and Name
3. Move and Breathe
4. Transform and Reframe

Say it out loud a few times – it's got a nice little rhythm and rhyme to help you remember it.

1. Stop and Notice

Observe what is happening for you physically, mentally and emotionally – e.g. you might have sweaty palms, a lump in your throat, negative and anxious thoughts, worries, nerves and "what ifs?".

At this stage, stop and simply notice. Watch your thoughts, let them come and go. No need to change anything.

You are pausing, making space and not rushing. You are preparing yourself. You are fine-tuning your awareness and ability to communicate well.

2. Acknowledge and Name

Begin acknowledging and naming or labelling your thoughts and feelings, e.g. "I'm feeling nervous" / "I'm feeling stressed" / "I'm excited" / "I'm wondering what I will do if this doesn't go well" / "What if what I say makes things worse?" / "I'm worried about what the other person will think/say/do."

You are switching on the more rational part of your brain.

3. Move and Breathe

Gently begin to move areas of your body. Wiggle your toes and your fingers, relax your jaw. Or press your hands together, scrunch your face or squeeze your knees up and down.

Loosening your body, unlocks your brain.

Notice your breathing, the rise and fall of your belly or chest. The cold air as you breathe in through your nostrils and the warmth as it moves around your body and out again. Stay with the in and out of your breath for a short while.

You're bringing yourself into your body and out of the chatter of your mind.

YOUR BREATH – YOUR GREATEST TOOL

I met Aicha McKenzie at our Pjoys launch. She was a gymnast, then a dancer and is now Founder of AMCK – a talent agency; she is also a Breath Work Coach. I love how she describes the simple benefits of using the breath as a tool and how it begins to work its best when you can weave it into the day-to-day of your life, treating it as something you can drop into when you feel that worry being manufactured, awkward emerging or anxiety rising. She explained:

I use the breath to trigger the stillness. It gives me the best chance to slow down my mind just enough for the chaos to start to make some sense. By consciously breathing in specific patterns, I can self-sufficiently bring down my heart rate and reset my nervous system to a level of chill, especially when it's feeling frantic and stressed. Coupled with using essential oils, my daily breath practice is my way into meditation. Sometimes I do it with music, other times in silence. Even when I get disturbed by my children or other things, I try to hold my own peace and continue to zone into myself. That's the practice ... Can you meditate and keep breathing deeply when "life" is doing its thing? It's not easy, but it is possible, and I practise this every day so that it becomes my default setting.

4. Transform and Reframe

Ask yourself transformative and compassionate questions and reframe how you think and feel about the situation:

- How can I grow from this experience?
- Do I have evidence for the awkward feelings, scenarios and responses I am imagining?
- Is this truly fear and danger?
- Am I manufacturing worry?
- How is the conversation I'm about to have kind and caring?
- Is this an opportunity to make the uncomfortable comfortable?
- I am feeling my feelings. This is natural.
- If I Own My Awkward, it will help the other person own theirs.
- I can make a positive difference by talking about mental health.

- I am ready to have a conversation.
- I care.

You are reframing your neural pathways and the way you're seeing the situation.

INDICATORS AND SIGNALS

Bryan Niederhelm, VP and Director of Threat Assessment and Management at Gavin de Becker Associates, has managed some of the US's most sensitive threat assessments involving some of the most well-known public figures and presidents. We chatted over several sessions about Gavin's ideas and Bryan's own insights. He told me:

When I reflect on the things that I'm most proud of, they are always the things that were hardest to do. For me, as soon as I feel a hesitation about doing something develop, I know now that it's an indicator to do it. A sign toward fulfilment. And so, I go for it. It happens more quickly and easily the more I practise it.

And so, with Bryan's unignorable inspiration and the Four Steps To Owning Your Awkward, let's practise tapping into those awkward signals, reframing the physical sensations of fear, owning the awkward pause, Owning *Our* Awkward and transforming panic into our power by pushing on through into the conversation. Think of it all like a strength training for our souls.

TRY THIS ...

We *all* have something that makes us feel awkward. What's yours? It can be anything, it doesn't have to be about mental health conversations.

What does it feel like? Look like? How does it show up? When you think about it, what's happening? What's the narrative or chitter-chatter in your head?

Practise using the Four Steps To Owning Your Awkward to reframe it and notice how you feel.

Use a notebook or journal to work through the steps or, if you prefer, talk them through with someone.

NAMING THE AWKWARD

Shanice Mears and I met through Livity. She is now the Co-founder of an inclusion agency called The Elephant Room. She brings to life the value of acknowledging and naming awkward feelings and demonstrates how, by asking herself transformative questions, she begins to reframe her awkward into something useful:

My sister was diagnosed with psychosis when I was ten years old and for almost ten years, I felt many things – ashamed, sad, confused, angry – and I never knew how to talk about it. In the past six years I've learned to navigate those conversations and I've learned that a lot of it starts with the conversation with yourself. I think I Own My Awkward by firstly admitting that it is awkward. I like to be upfront about stuff, so I'll just say it head on, that way there are no elephants in the room (pun intended). I don't blame myself for things anymore. I've turned blame into accountability and if things don't go well, I ask myself "What is this teaching me?" instead of being angry at myself for making a mistake.

REFRAMING THOSE PHYSICAL SENSATIONS FOR GOOD

When we are nervous, fearful, stressed, embarrassed and awkward, we often experience physical sensations that accompany all the unhelpful thoughts racing through our minds.

Wouldn't it be great to activate them to your advantage? To view them as signals that you are present and that you have the opportunity to do something good and useful? Let's reframe them.

Heart rate: In Flight and Fight your heart beats faster to bring oxygen to your major muscles. In Freeze, your heart rate might increase or decrease.
Reframe: You are alive. You HAVE a heart, and this is an opportunity to activate the compassionate part of it.

Lungs: In Flight and Fight your breathing speeds up to deliver more oxygen to your blood. In Freeze, you might hold your breath or restrict breathing.
Reframe: This is your REMINDER to breathe and enter the Four Steps To Owning Your Awkward.

Eyes: In Flight and Fight your peripheral vision increases so you can notice your surroundings. Your pupils dilate and let in more light, which helps you see better.
Reframe: This is the opportunity to truly connect and give someone your full attention.

Ears: In Flight and Fight your ears "perk up" and your hearing becomes sharper.
Reframe: All the better for listening, really listening with.

Hands and feet: As blood flow increases to your major muscles, your hands and feet might get cold.
Reframe: Cold feet? It's natural to want to avoid the conversation, but you can do this. Own Your Awkward and go for it.

SWEATY KNICKERS

Speaking of physical responses to stressful situations ... Lara Morgan is an experienced and voracious entrepreneur, business leader and mentor, who started her first business, Pacific Direct, at the age of 23 and sold it 17 years later for £20 million. So, when she offers an insight, I take notice. I've included it here as it's another useful sign and signal of when your body is responding to nerves, uncertainty and the awkward in all kinds of ways etc. I enjoy the way Laura champions the case for pushing yourself into the uncomfortable as often as you can. NB: you might need to stock up on undies. She told me:

I find myself smiling at the endless fabulous outcomes and wonderful experiences that have come about because, throughout my life, I have chosen to get surprisingly comfortable with being uncomfortably challenged. I call these "sweaty knickered moments". Those times when I push myself to try new things, taste differently, go to scary places, but mostly have conversations that are outside my comfort zone. I have practised becoming more able to crack on and try. Despite not knowing, often hoping (sometimes praying), I have been telling myself that the outcome, the progress, whether good or great (possibly bad), is still progress worth trying for and always better than not having a go.

FIND THE *FREE* IN *REFRAME*

So, with great knowledge and the foundations in place, we're ready to access and activate our natural ability to transform and reframe the negative into the positive. There's a free in reframe, can you see it? Like so many things in life, when you can see it, you can be it.

If awkward is unwieldy and unco-ordinated, the talking frameworks SENSE (see Chapter 5) and BRAVE (see Chapter 7) will give you the grace and elegance to embrace it. If awkward is nerves, you now know they are there because you care and we're going to channel them in the most wonderful of ways. Awkward doesn't have to stay tricky, it doesn't have to be labelled as a threat, it can represent courage and bravery, action and asking.

Awkward is kindness about to happen.

LOVE

I'm not quite sure how to do justice to the role my husband plays in supporting me in my story now, and in the most difficult of times. He was my Personal Survival Kit during that episode of burnout, depression and anxiety, my anchor, but before and after that time he has been the most incredible partner in love and life. I share wholeheartedly the reflection of the legendary Ruth Bader Ginsburg, who so sadly died in 2020: "To have a caring life partner, you help the other person when that person needs it. I had a life partner who thought my work was as important as his, and I think that made all the difference to me."

Remi fed and watered me, kept me safe, brought beauty into my life and all with a kindness and non-judgement that came, not from any training, but from a place of love. I don't find it easy to ask for help, but I can at least accept it from Remi, if a little awkwardly.

He is a talented artist and incredibly motivated and hard-working, his work selling all over the world. He is also one of the friendliest and upbeat artists around, with an amazing skill of connecting with others. He is the extrovert to my introvert and I would in no way describe him as a stereotypical "tortured" artist, yet I was touched to be reminded of the fragility within us all and the impact that judgemental language and opinions, yet again, can have on our mental health and wellbeing when I talked to him about awkward moments:

As an artist I often have ups and downs. There's a huge amount of work, investment and energy, both physical and mental that goes into creating a body of work for an exhibition. You open the exhibition with hope, expectation and excitement and after the show has opened, regardless of how much work has sold and how many people tell you they loved it, there is nearly always a dip. I have spoken to so many of my artist friends who describe the exact same feelings. Why do we do it to ourselves you may ask? Maybe it's the need for appreciation, the want of success or maybe it's just because we all love what we do and want so much for other people to feel and connect with it.

I remember a time when a gallery asked me to drop by for a chat. On first impressions the people I met seemed very nice and professional, so it took me back when they began to break down exactly what they thought was wrong with my work. I didn't know how to reply. One of them even told me that without a recognized art education I would never be taken seriously. Maybe what I should have said was that I had exhibited my work in museums in Spain, Singapore, France, and more, and had recently spoken at Tate Modern, or that I had exhibited and painted murals all over the world, but I didn't. I was embarrassed, feeling awkward and like a complete imposter.

I left, unable to stand up for myself, my work or my career and I felt utterly crushed. How they made me feel lasted and I spent the following weeks after the meeting feeling entirely worthless and considered jacking my art career in and giving up making art forever. I realized just how fragile my mental state could be and after a period of reflection, a break from making art and talking about how I was feeling with people I trusted, I made a vow to myself to never let that happen again.

I still think back to that conversation and how easy it is to set someone on the road to potentially experiencing a huge dip in their mental health, by criticizing them and pulling them apart. We are all human and I make it a point to never do that to other people because I know all too well how it made me feel. I Own My Awkward by being true to myself and trying to remember that no one is better or worse than anyone else. Keeping that in mind helps me see others as an equal and that those awkward conversations, moments and feelings are going on for them as much as for me.

FROM AWKWARD TO AWESOME!

Are you ready? It's time. Put on the T-shirt (or your PJs of course) and say it out loud ...

The Awkward Promise

I (insert name here) am ready to step into the space of awkward and stay there.

I will feel my nerves, I will hold my nerve, I will stop and notice the awkward pause and thoughts. I'll acknowledge and name them and activate the rational part of my brain. I'll gently move and breathe, getting out of my head, into my body so that I can remind myself that what I'm about to do is in service and kindness to either myself or to someone else, and that either way, that is awesome not awkward. I'll be curious and ask myself transformative and compassionate questions that will reframe my fear and set me up for a brave conversation. I know it is easier to turn away, I also know it is better to push on through the awkward and start the conversation.

So, here I go, into the unknown response, ready for my cheeks to sting, my heart to beat a little faster, I'm going to use that extra energy to help me Own My Awkward, knowing that if I Own My Awkward, it will help the person I'm about to talk to own theirs.

I'm ready to make a difference. I'm ready to help myself if I am asking for help and to help someone else if I'm offering help.

Signed (insert name here)

THE CORNERSTONES OF AWKWARD CONVERSATIONS

Confidence

If you weren't there already, this is the moment you can truly begin to Own Your Awkward and once you begin your confidence will grow and grow.

Capability

Put the Four Steps To Owning Your Awkward into your toolkit: Stop and Notice, Acknowledge and Name, Move and Breathe, Transform and Reframe.

Communication

Pick up on the physical sensations your body is using to communicate with you and activate them to your advantage.

Compassion

Thích Nhất Hạnh is a Vietnamese Thiền Buddhist monk and peace activist and has been referred to as "The Father of Mindfulness". He describes compassion as a verb, something we should be doing. So let's stop waiting for it to arrive and instead work on building it within ourselves. By reaching the end of this chapter, you are developing your ability to do it.

CHAPTER 5

The SENSE Framework: Helping Someone

"You may not always have a comfortable life and you will not always be able to solve all of the world's problems at once, but don't ever underestimate the importance you can have because history has shown us that courage can be contagious and hope can take on a life of its own."

Michelle Obama

I've found that most people find it far easier to join the awkward movement by improving their confidence and skills for *offering* someone help, to support someone struggling with *their* mental health and wellbeing, rather than to help *themselves*, and to *ask* for help when *they* need it. It's far easier to give to others than ourselves, right? Remember Give Give Get? That's why I'm starting by giving you the SENSE framework to help you help others. Let's say I'm easing you in, but do get ready to learn how to ask for help for yourself by using the BRAVE framework (see Chapter 7). Trust me when I say you can't be great at one without the other.

Humans are generally good, better than good mostly, and I assume that if you are reading this book, you are one of those better than good humans with all the right intentions. I'm taking a confident guess that you are kind and thoughtful and primarily motivated to help others and be part of this awkward movement, to make talking about our mental health easier, everyday chat. The compassion is already within you – the SENSE framework is here to help unlock it and let it do its best. It will give you increased confidence and capability around the common sense and natural instincts you already have.

TWO DAYS THAT TRANSFORMED MY LIFE

When I began telling my story of mental ill-health publicly, in 2017, just as Pjoys was taking shape and gaining momentum, I quickly felt the positive impact and power of sharing. People began to share back their experiences of poor mental health with me, either their own or that of someone they knew; sometimes past, sometimes present.

Whilst I was feeling more of an expert on my own mental health, I wasn't prepared for the amount of personal disclosure I was receiving from people who had read articles I had written, who I met in and out of work, or who were in the audience or groups of my mental health talks and sessions. Although I could feel my mission rising in impact, I became increasingly concerned that I was not fully equipped to respond in the right and most confident way to people telling me about their mental health. I felt I needed to be better equipped and so I started searching for some training that was accessible, relatively speedy and robust.

I quickly found a two-day course called Mental Health First Aid (MHFA) training, which turned out to be utterly transformational. The knowledge, confidence and framework for supporting someone with their mental health, especially in a crisis, that I came away with felt empowering and so very useful, and I found myself putting it into practice almost immediately, with a great sense of relief and gratitude for having these new skills. I also discovered it was an invaluable and ongoing way to continue to understand, protect and look after my own mental health and recovery.

I love a bit of professional and personal development and most of mine had been rooted in business and leadership training. I learned so much from the two days of training – it felt brilliantly aligned to the new direction and space I was finding my voice in, with Pjoys and my public speaking, so much so that I applied to do the MHFA England Instructor training. It should be noted at this point, if you haven't picked it up already, I'm a kind of "all or nothing" type of human, which is mostly a blessing, occasionally a burden and often exhausting!

FIRST AID TRAINING

Danielle Bridge is the CEO of a First Aid Training Social Enterprise and we trained to become MHFA Instructors together. Through her Social Enterprise she also delivers physical first aid training and so is perfectly placed to share a view on the importance of mental versus physical first aid:

Physical first aid has been around for a long time – we are used to the language, the narrative and the expectation on the public and first aiders alike. Mental ill-health, however, is scary, unknown, and far too complex for us to be able to help as the average non-medical person, right?

The aim of physical first aid is to preserve life, prevent deterioration and promote recovery.

MHFA is pretty much the same, with the aim being to provide comfort and support to a person living with mental ill-health or in a crisis, by providing understanding, active listening and signposting. This early recognition and help can truly be as lifesaving as physical first aid interventions. Having a better understanding of our capabilities as a human being to help another human being means we can have a greater impact on the lives of others.

So, one is no more important than the other and they can both save lives? Good to know.

Mental Health First Aid (MHFA) International oversees 26 accredited MHFA Programmes in 24 countries worldwide, with over 4 million Mental Health First Aiders trained across the globe since its inception in 2000, including Michelle Obama!

MHFA England's ambition is to get 1 in 10 of the UK workforce trained as Mental Health First Aiders. It's an ambitious target, but by no means unattainable and it's an important goal to strive for. We'll know real change has happened when we get there. And we will get there!

FEEDER FRAMEWORKS

A year or so into teaching MHFA, I found myself wondering about all the people who want to feel confident supporting people struggling with their mental health, but for whom MHFA training isn't possible. Through my work I could *feel* the need. Beyond the MHFA training I was offering, I wondered how I could better support those who feel nervous about starting a conversation about mental health, because of all those fears, concerns and awkwardness. How could I help as many people as possible feel confident and have a starting point to talk about mental health in work, schools, colleges and universities, at home, while socializing and in our communities?

I also found myself wondering how we could help more people have greater awareness of their own poor mental health if it develops and encourage them to act and ask for support when needed, as early on as possible. Essentially, how could I help more people have the courage to ask for help?

Inspired by speaking to hundreds of people about both mine and their experiences and stories of mental ill-health, I created the SENSE and BRAVE talking frameworks. I like to think of them as "feeder frameworks" for MHFA training, because I believe that most people would benefit from taking part in the MHFA course. I do, however, recognize that not everyone is quite ready for or has the time or resources to do MHFA right now. So, these talking frameworks provide a starting point.

THE SENSE FRAMEWORK

Safety – Create a safe space to have a conversation.
Empathy – Let them talk. Truly listen. Connect.
Non-judgement – It's not about you. Accept their experience.
Support – Let them know they are not alone.
Encouragement – Gently encourage them to seek help.

Common Sense

Why SENSE? Because when I'm leading mental health training sessions, I find that people soon begin to realize that much of having a conversation about mental health is about applying the common sense they already have. If you then add a great big sprinkle of confidence by building and improving your knowledge, as well as adding to your capability with a simple framework or two, then you really are good to go. So, let's look at the framework of SENSE in a little more detail.

S for Safety
Create a safe space to start a conversation.

- Tell them you are here to listen, that you care.
- When can you make time to talk to them? Ensure you have time for a decent chat (if they want).
- Where would the best place be to make them feel comfortable? Perhaps invite them for a walk/coffee/juice/phone call/Zoom call? Give them options, choice and control, which might even be communicating by text or email initially.
- Minimize background noise and activity – you want to create a good flow, or for it to be okay to be quiet.
- In an emergency, seek support depending upon the circumstances and remember you are not the mental health professional (unless of course you actually are!). Get help.

E for Empathy
Let them talk. Truly listen. Connect.

- Seek to understand their pain. Acknowledge and connect.
- Think about your body language and avoid being in any way "confrontational" – sitting side by side at a slight angle is likely to be more comfortable than sitting directly opposite one another. Walking is a great alternative, if the person would like to do that.
- Use indicators, such as nods, mmms, yes, to let them know you are truly listening.

- Don't feel like you must give a response or suggestion to everything they say. Listening, truly listening, might be the greatest gift you can give them (see Chapter 6 for how to do this effectively).
- Use your Frame of Reference and Life Footprint (see page 48) to find commonalities and empathically feel their challenges.

N for Non-judgement
It's not about you. Accept their experience.

- You're not here to judge right or wrong.
- Remember, judgement can be conveyed physically as well as verbally. Be aware of your body language, your expressions, your concentration and attention, your tone.
- Try your best to understand, but accept you might not. You can still support them. Accept the person and what they are sharing as their truth at that moment.
- Remember, we are all different. Our Frame of Reference is what shapes our views, behaviours and our responses come from a lifetime of experiences unique to each of us – our unique Life Footprint.
- Notice and acknowledge your feelings; you can't stop them coming, but you can choose to put them to one side.

S for Support
Let them know they are not alone.

- Ask if there is anything that they think might help. Offer additional ideas that might be helpful if you have them. Remember, don't tell, offer.

- Find ways to reassure them without diminishing what they are experiencing.
- Normalize what they are experiencing, feeling and thinking – i.e. it's more common than you might think for people to struggle with their mental health and wellbeing and there is help you can get.
- Let them know they are not alone. Let them know that you care.
- Let them know that there is always hope and that recovery is the most likely outcome.

E for Encouragement
Gently encourage them to seek help.

- Let them know they're brave for talking about how they are feeling.
- Have they spoken to anyone already? If they have, ask them what helped then? What was useful?
- Let them know that there are lots of different types of professional help. You might be able to signpost them toward that help (see Useful Resources).
- Encourage them to speak to their doctor or another mental health professional and reassure them they won't be wasting anyone's time.
- Beyond your conversation, encourage them to keep talking, either to you and/or others.

Remember, this is a framework to guide you rather than a rigid set of rules, so adapt it as you need to. It's a little bit like a sat nav with several routes you can take to get to your destination.

Some routes will be quicker than others, some more scenic, sometimes you'll suddenly find yourself at a standstill, in a traffic jam, occasionally there might be a bump in the road; some journeys are joyful, some are not, but remember, you'll often have the option to change route, and try a different way. The journey might not be perfect, but if we just keep going we nearly always get to where we are heading in the end. It's the same with conversations.

INTUITION – EXPLORING A HUNCH

In my conversation with Bryan Niederhelm (see page 83), I discovered a number of golden threads of humanity running through GDBA and his leadership, in particular his three Cs – Care, Compassion and Curiosity. Remember, this is a business about protection, security and managing threats (read people) of the most serious nature. Bryan explained that 50% of his energy is invested in managing client fear and that by encouraging people to adopt a sense of compassion for someone or something they fear, they are able to think more rationally, which means they become calmer and are better placed to truly hear Bryan and his team, take direction and, as a result, employ better safety strategies. What if we took Bryan's compassionate approach to fear management and applied it to the awkward moments we find ourselves in, to create a calmer, more rational place from which to have better conversations? *The Four Steps To Owning Your Awkward step in from stage right*.

Bryan helped me better understand some of the aspects of Gavin de Becker's book, *The Gift of Fear*, – not just about the role of fear but also the role of intuition. This gave credence to a hunch I had been playing with and, which if I'm honest, I'd not been too sure of including in my SENSE framework for fear (or more like manufactured worry?) of stepping too much into an "alternative" space. I love most things alternative by the way – in fact complementary and aligned are far better descriptors – but I had a niggle alongside the hunch that including intuition might make the framework feel less robust. Turns out my hunch was stronger than my niggle and intuition became a firm feature in my SENSE framework.

SENSE becomes *SENSES*

Introducing my magic sixth letter, S, for Sixth Sense. It's there to remind us of the power of our intuition, our gut feelings and instincts and our "Spidey" senses. If something doesn't *feel* right, act and ask. You know those times, when you can't put your finger on what or why, but you just have a feeling that there's "something". In these moments there is a good chance your intuition is at work and has picked something up. In my conversation with Bryan, he reminded me that our intuition's only goal is to protect us and is best described as knowing or understanding something immediately based on our feelings rather than facts. An in-built survival mechanism, our activated intuition is always in response to something and always has our best interests at heart. So, when we are tapped into our intuition, we are more open to and aware of the signs and signals giving us subtle, almost undetectable, but perhaps important, information.

Let's consider the outcomes of asking someone if they are okay because you are responding to your intuition. If it turns out there is something wrong, by asking you will have created an open door for someone to start talking about how they are feeling. A gift of kindness and care! And if there's nothing wrong, well brilliant, it's no less a gift of care and concern, is it? Are they going to feel offended that you asked if they are okay? Unlikely. Better still, perhaps by showing you care and are not afraid to ask and talk about how someone is feeling, they'll know you are someone they can talk to if they ever need to in the future. There's also the chance that you ask and they say that nothing's wrong, but there is. Your intuition was right, but you can't make someone tell you what's wrong and they will still leave that conversation feeling your kindness and care and, when ready, perhaps you'll be the person they feel able to talk to – and don't forget, you can always check back in and ask again.

S for Sixth Sense
Listen to your gut feeling.
- Listen to your intuition. If in doubt, act and ask.
- If you have a feeling or sense that something's not right, there's a good chance you are right.
- Sometimes we get a niggle, a feeling; it's easy to dismiss it, feel like we are misinterpreting something or that it's not our business, not our place, but maybe that feeling stays with us, or keeps coming back. Listen to it and take notice of it.

- What are you noticing? What are the signals and the signs that something is up?
- Once you've asked, drop into the SENSE framework from the top.

Make the time, have that conversation, ask explicitly if someone is doing okay. It could make all the difference. Get SENSES working even harder as you tap into your senses beyond intuition. Hearing, feeling and seeing can all give you clues, signs and signals that someone needs support.

Your New Best Frenemies?

Responding to your intuition isn't about following a checklist, but as Gavin says, "Unlike worry, it won't waste your time, it will send you messengers to get your attention." In the broad ranking of Gavin's "Messengers of Intuition", the one with the greatest urgency is fear – always listen to it. The next level is apprehension, then suspicion, hesitation, doubt, gut feelings and hunches and curiosity. Nagging feelings, persistent thoughts, physical sensations, wonder and anxiety are less urgent in terms of immediate danger, but perhaps play a more important role when it comes to picking up clues about someone's mental health. Indicators all around, are discomfort and unease our New Best Frenemies?

And then there's humour, a more surprising messenger, but one that should be taken seriously in terms of being alert to fear and danger and one that, when you stop to think about it, makes sense in terms of the many people who manage or even cover up their poor mental health through the use of humour.

Bryan agreed that "awkward" could sit quite (un)comfortably alongside the other Messengers of Intuition. Who would have thought that the world's leading experts on violent behaviour would be the endorsers for the sixth sense in my SENSE talking framework?

In summary, if you find yourself thinking "it's probably nothing", it might be your greatest signal to ask someone if everything is okay.

GETTING IN *THE* RIGHT STATE, NOT *A* RIGHT STATE

Sometimes you will find yourself in a conversation about mental health with perhaps little or no notice, and at other times you'll want to start a conversation because you are concerned about someone and will have longer to think about and prepare for it. Either way your awkward is probably kicking in and now is a good time to use the Four Steps To Owning Your Awkward (see page 80). Remember, you're doing all of this to help someone. You are amazing. Awkward yes, but you're super amazing as well.

Conversation Starters

Okay, so you've Owned Your Awkward using the Four Steps (see Chapter 4), now how do you start the conversation? Argh. Blank page, blank mind. Where to begin? This is where some preparation and useful opening lines are handy. This is an exercise worth adding to, personalizing and tucking into your toolkit. It's good to say some of these conversation starters out loud, perhaps even add your own tone. You want to sound like you after all.

- "I wanted to check in with you and see if everything's okay?"
- "How are you *today*?"
- "You've been on my mind."
- "It seems like it's been a stressful time for you. How are you doing?"
- "I've noticed that … you've not been around/you've been working late/you don't seem yourself."
- "I just wanted to let you know that I'm here for you if you'd like to talk."
- "What would you like to talk about today?"
- "How can I support you right now?"
- "Fancy a chat/walk?" (sometimes keeping it simple is best)
- "How's everyone showing up?" (Group conversations can be good for getting a sense of how individuals are. I would lead the beginning of our Livity leadership team meetings by asking this question, often starting with how I was feeling to help set the tone and permission to speak freely – and you might create a "That's Me'" moment for someone).

CONVERSATION NON-STARTERS

You might recognize some of the phrases below; you might have even said some of them. This is not the time to beat yourself up if you have, but an opportunity to shift your language and approach. We're all a work in progress. These really are conversation *non-starters*, they can only serve to shout stigma, shame, embarrassment, worthlessness, drama, disregard and disbelief.

- "Cheer up, it might never happen."
- "Why the long face?"
- "Chin up."
- "You're lucky, look at everything you have in your life."
- "Look on the bright side."
- "Things could be worse."
- "There are people much worse off than you."
- "Let's look at the positives."
- "You know what you should do ..."
- "It's a bit awkward when you talk about your mental health."

Keeping the Conversation Going

Brilliant, you've Owned Your Awkward and started the conversation. Whoop and well done!

But where is it going? Well, none of us really know. What we do know is one of the most difficult aspects of talking about mental health has been conquered. Now we want to play our part in keeping the conversation going. Below are some "keeping it going" lines that you might want to use as a starting point, but phrase in a way that suits you (try to make most of your statements and questions open where possible, as opposed to questions that can only be answered with a yes/no closed response):

- "I hear you. How does that make you feel?"
- "That sounds tough. Can you tell me more?"
- "Who else have you spoken to about how you are feeling? (or "Who could you speak to?" if they say no one).
- "It's really brave of you to share how you are feeling. How can I help?"
- "Can you tell me more about that?"
- "How long have you felt like this?"
- "Would you feel comfortable telling me more?"
- "Thank you for telling me. How can I support you?"
- "What else have you been experiencing?"
- "What are the things that are helpful or useful when you feel like this? What's unhelpful?"

TRAUMA

Amanda May Daly is a photographer and pal and I'm grateful to her for sharing her experience of trauma. She reminds us that those of us who have our own experiences of mental ill-health, are often uniquely placed to provide an ear and a whole lot of hope to someone experiencing their own challenges. We really are the cheerleaders and front runners of the Own Your Awkward message. She told me:

There is an advice column in New York Magazine called "Ask Polly" and there was a letter from a woman who got dumped, fired and found out she probably couldn't have children pretty much all at once. The response to that letter was long and beautiful but what has always really stuck with me was that "Polly" pointed out that once you have been crushed under life's Wheel of Fortune you are in a much better position to be a good friend to other people who feel like their world is ending. I have personally found this to be so true. The trauma I endured in childhood and the coping mechanisms I developed because of that trauma were a crash course in developing a unique brand of sensitivity and empathy that make me who I am today. I am so glad that I am trauma aware because the reality is that trauma exists in a spectrum across the human experience and those of us who have endured it and survived can choose to be a lifeline and a harbinger of hope for others along the way. So, whether it's the death of a child's pet, a friend leaving an abusive relationship or someone having mental health issues, I know that I can be of service, just by being me, because I know what it's like to feel lower than low and still rise above.

TRY THIS ...

Using the SENSE framework is the best way to, well, start using it. You might be a little nervous, perhaps shy, and definitely awkward, but give it a go. You have the Four Steps To Owning Your Awkward in Chapter 4, the SENSE framework in this chapter, as well as the conversation tips and guides on pages 106–109.

- Begin by saying some of these words, questions and conversation starters and ideas out loud; hearing yourself saying them will remove the first layer of the awkward onion.
- Ask someone you trust if you can practise on them/ with them. If you want to role play and give more of a mental health story to your practising, imagine your friend has been less communicative lately. You can't put your finger on it; they just don't seem themselves. They've been taking quite a bit of time off work with illness, for different reasons, and they've dropped out of the last couple of social occasions.
- Use SENSE to practise how you might talk to them.

Once you've finished, using a notebook or journal or just talking through with your role-play partner, reflect on what came easily and comfortably. What felt more challenging and would benefit from more thought and practice?

When the Conversation Doesn't Go Well

There are going to be conversations that don't go well for all kinds of reasons. Sometimes it's not the right timing for the other person. Sometimes the person may be defensive, embarrassed, emotional and the same might even happen to you. You might say something unhelpful; it happens. Until we are actually in the conversation we can only imagine what might not go well and, remember, worry is manufactured and shouldn't get in the way of Owning Your Awkward and asking someone how they are. When a conversation doesn't go well, try using these ideas to keep you moving forward:

- Create time and space to reflect, even if it feels uncomfortable.
- Can you pinpoint where it didn't go so well?
- Where did it go well?
- Remember, you started the conversation to be of help. Go easy on yourself.
- Do you need to say sorry for anything that, on reflection, you said or didn't say?
- If you are mid-conversation and if it feels like it's not going well, could it be useful to suggest a short break from talking to get some space and reset?
- It might be that you're not the best person for this conversation. Ask them who might be.
- Try not to ruminate.
- Don't be afraid to come back to the conversation. Ask permission to start again.
- Acknowledge your awkward; it may help them acknowledge theirs.

THE AWKWARDNESS OF NOT KNOWING

Sian Anderson is a DJ and presenter on BBC Radio 1Xtra and we have been friends since our Livity days. Sian identifies another kind of awkward that is well worth sharing, as we've probably all been there. That moment when we become aware that someone else's mental health challenges have been going on for a while and feel terrible that we hadn't picked up on it or that the person hadn't felt able to tell us until now. Awkward can hijack you in so many sneaky ways. She told me:

I've felt uncomfortable that someone close to me could be struggling and suffering in silence, but putting a smile on their face publicly for months. It feels like a huge relief when they speak to me about it. I just try to be present, be understanding and listen, which, as someone who wants to fix everyone and everything, can be awkward because I want to make them feel better immediately, but I know now to be patient and just be there for them.

You might benefit from using the Four Steps To Owning Your Awkward in this situation, rather than remaining in the unproductive place of feeling bad, sad and mad with yourself for not knowing. Reframe: you are here now, and they are telling you how they feel. Like Sian, be patient, Own Your Awkward, so they can own theirs, and drop into the SENSE framework.

Conversation Watch-Outs

Ever since I've had a better understanding of the topic of mental health, alongside feeling far better informed about and protective of my own, I've felt more confident, capable and clear about my role in supporting someone with their mental health. A couple of lessons that were initially surprising to me, and I now view as invaluable reminders, I gift to you here. Let's call it fast-tracking your framework induction:

- Avoid trying to fix or give solutions. It's not your job.
- Remember we are all different, we each have our unique Life Footprint. No judging.
- It's unlikely you know "exactly" how someone feels. So, try not to say it.
- Be aware of hurrying someone to get to the point. Give them the time they need.
- Whilst you want to help create a safe and confidential space, never agree to keeping suicidal thinking or planning secret.
- Try your best to use helpful and non-stigmatizing language.
- Avoid comparing the person's situation to someone else's or your own.
- Be mindful to not make the person feel guilty – e.g. telling someone to "think of" their family might just add to their negative feelings about themselves.
- Take on board everything about listening in the next chapter.
- It can be useful to reference your own experience to help someone feel less alone; just don't make it all about you.

UNLOCKING EMPATHY

Nihal Arthanayake is a journalist and presenter, and a friend of my husband Remi. I first met him on what must have been my second or third date with Remi. There was an awkwardly joyful moment when we arrived at a club, where Remi and Nihal, both very cool, got on the dance floor immediately. I'm just not a "get on the dance floor as quickly as possible" kind of gal – I need to build up to it – so with my social anxiety screaming, it got worse before it got better. Remi did some kind of moonwalk across the dance floor – I can't remember if Nihal was also moonwalking, but I do remember they were both brilliant and joyfully free dancers, which made my heart sink and sing at the same time. The fact that these days I dance around the kitchen (and occasionally other dance floors) freely and joyfully is more proof that awkward can be overcome. Nihal told me:

I talk to strangers for a living about the most intimate parts of their lives, from a mother who lost her son to the Syrian regime to a former sex worker who had endured years of abuse. These conversations can have a profound effect on me, and I have been known to shed more than a tear or two when listening to stories that involved heartache and trauma. In order to empathize, you have to open up a space within yourself with the door wide open. That is both positive and negative. I feel that I can express my sadness to the world. Sharing it helps me.

Nihal talks about finding and opening up a space within himself in order to unlock empathy. You can do it too – remember, you have your Frame of Reference, the story of you and all that contributes to your Life Footprint. Within your story sit moments and experiences that will help you connect to someone else's pain or hurt, even if you haven't experienced or been affected by something in a similar way. Plus, you have your imagination and this is where it might come in useful.

FEELING SEEN AND HEARD

Mentors come in many different shapes, sizes and, in the case of Bejay Mulenga, ages. Bejay is the Founder of Supa Network and we have known each other for well over a decade. We met through a Livity project. Bejay was 14, and already running his first enterprise, Supa Tuck, *in* school, whilst still *at* school, and I was *mumbles 39* and running Livity. I like to think we were one of the first successful blueprints for "two-way mentoring". Bejay's enthusiasm and ambition were infectious from the first time we said hello and have been ever since. He told me:

Establishing intimacy and focusing on building a rela-tionship with the person, or the people we are engaging with is key. When sharing vulnerability, especially around mental health, it's important to ensure people feel like they are being heard and seen. Really spending time sharing information about yourself, and encouraging the people around you to do the same, is the perfect precursor to a conversation about mental health. It doesn't have to be super loaded or heavy – just authentic and personal, to set the scene and tone.

I really love the idea of doing your best to ensure the person you are talking to feels both seen and heard and in the next chapter I'm going to share with you my most treasured tactic for helping you achieve it.

THE CORNERSTONES OF AWKWARD CONVERSATIONS

Confidence
Having a conversation is often about using your common sense.

Capability
You now have the SENSE framework. Have a go at using it.

Communication
Intuition is real. If you have a gut feeling, listen to it. Act. Ask.

Compassion
Empathy over sympathy every time. Use your Frame of Reference and your Life Footprint to unlock the compassionate space within you.

CHAPTER 6

The Power of the Pause

"The most called-upon prerequisite of a friend is an accessible ear."

Maya Angelou

Before we move on to the next framework, let's take a moment to reflect, to rest, to recover, to give the information, ideas and, I hope, a little inspiration the space to bubble, absorb and land. This chapter is dedicated to valuing the importance of communication, the cornerstone that supports both the delivery and receipt of all those awkward offers of, and asks for, help. Conversations, like music and songs, have rhythm, they have tone, they can be fast, slow, soft, loud. Some are long, some short, some leave you feeling joyful, some calm, others flat. Some we love, others not so much. Some have words and lyrics, others don't and yet can be as, if not more, powerful. Sometimes we are performing them, sometimes we join in and often we are simply listening to them.

Ah, listening, so powerful, yet often underrated, undervalued and not always so well understood.

There is a beautiful conversation tactic that I have learned to use and that I adore and depend upon, not only in mental health conversations, but all conversations. It takes some practice and discipline and might even feel counterintuitive at first, awkward even, but I guess we're getting used to that by this part of the book. It's a thought, an idea, a strategy and a general reminder for life that I think you're going to like. It's ...

Wait for it ...

Wait ...

Hold on ...

Just a moment longer ...

And here it is ... the pause.

"What made the biggest difference was when someone truly listened to me" isn't one person's quote, it's what many of the people I've spoken to about mental health conversations tell me. They'll describe how, once they finally felt able to talk about how they were feeling and when they were being given time, space and attention to share, they experienced a great sense of being truly listened to, and how that was so valuable. Sounds so small and obvious, doesn't it? But think about it, be honest – when was the last time you truly listened (or were truly listened to?), with 100% of your full attention, to someone else, with not one moment where your mind wandered, or your attention shifted elsewhere? There's a chance you may *think* you're a good listener, but I challenge you to spend a while reflecting on how you listen, how *well* you listen. This chapter is about talking less, listening more, listening better.

BEING HUMAN

As humans we naturally fill the silence when in conversation. We can't help ourselves! We chatter on and on. What you will discover here is that not being afraid of silence is powerful. Embracing silence is a gift, to you the listener, giving you time to craft a thoughtful and meaningful response, and it gives the person talking permission to go at their pace and find the way they want to talk, when they are ready to.

Another human trait is that when someone begins to talk to us, about almost anything, our attention is pulled away from the words they are speaking almost immediately. It's almost impossible to prevent. It's what our minds do. So, what's going on? All kinds of things!

- We might be thinking about how we are going to respond to what we are hearing.
- It could be that we have dropped straight into thinking about finding a solution or an offer of help and, as we learned in the previous chapter, that's not necessarily what someone needs from us.
- We may be wondering and worrying (remember, it's a manufactured fear and a waste of time) about getting

our response right or wrong, or we might find ourselves caught up in thinking about our own lives and experiences because of what we're hearing.

- It could easily be, although embarrassing to admit perhaps, that our mind has wandered completely away from the person talking, into our own world and to thoughts that have nothing to do with the conversation.
- Worse still, we could be having an uncomfortable response to what we are hearing; we might be experiencing judgemental or critical feelings.
- We might just not understand, and we've possibly found ourselves back in that awkward space again – argh, you've got to be kidding me? Well, no, no kidding, we are going to find ourselves back in the awkward space time and time again. The good news is that if you are experiencing any of that, it means you are having conversations and all that practising means you're getting really good at Owning Your Awkward.

It can be surprisingly hard to listen and to listen well – it takes practice and effort – but it is within us and it's worth becoming aware of, because it really could make the greatest difference to someone.

SILENCE IS GOLDEN

You've just asked someone how they are, or if everything is okay. You might have even been a little more explicit and told someone that you feel concerned for them and their mental health. This is brilliant – you've asked, you've acted, YES! Maybe you've used the SENSE framework to help you prepare for and navigate your way into and through a conversation, WHOOP! If you have, you are amazing and awesome and you are owning it, owning the uncomfortable, Owning Your Awkward.

And then what happens? Well, there's a good chance you might be met either immediately, or at some point mid-conversation, with what feels like an almighty LOUD silence. A great big, awkward gaping silence ... maybe an even bigger awkward than the one you were feeling and fighting with before you asked anything at all.

Let's think about it, reframe it even. Let's get into the other person's shoes for a moment. There's a good chance they might be about to share their thoughts and feelings for the first time, they may be about to talk about some of the deepest, most private, aspects of themselves, they're very likely trying to find the words, the language and the courage to explain what they are experiencing. They may be working out where on earth to start, how much to say or not say to you. They could be trying to compose themselves. There have been many times when I've been asked if I'm okay ... only for me to start welling up and feeling my emotions ten times harder *because* I've been asked how I am. It's that moment of release and relief when someone has made the brave decision to share what's happening for them or is touched that someone is showing genuine interest and concern, that can take someone by surprise. Let's face it, it's quite hard to talk with a great big lump in your throat, hence the silence.

Sit with the Silence

So how to respond to the silence?

- Firstly, don't feel any urgency to "keep calm and carry on" and keep the conversation going to avoid the awkward (we don't avoid that anymore, do we?).
- As best you can, reflect the quiet for a moment, mirror it, or maybe offer a short, helpful extension to your question. For example, "I was wondering how you are at the moment?" – *silence*. "I've noticed that you've not been around as much" – *silence*.
- Now HOLD the silence and space. This is you providing time and space for the words to come, for the person to find the best place to start or for their emotions to rise and fall. Be okay in the silence. As with awkward, if you are okay with the silence, it makes it easier for the other person to be okay with the silence.
- Enjoy and value the quiet and let them use it to find the best way for them to express themselves in their own words and in their own time. It takes practice and holding your nerve (and Owning Your Awkward), but it's going to be okay.

NO EXPERIENCE NECESSARY

Jess Butcher is an entrepreneur and business adviser. I've loved how we've evolved from having business exchanges to sharing more personal conversations over the years. Jess identifies the awkwardness of feeling inexperienced to talk about someone's mental health and what to do when it happens:

I have most definitely experienced the "awkward conversation" with regards to poor mental health with both close friends, family members and people I've managed who have experienced serious anxiety and depression. I've felt a little helpless as, whilst I've certainly had difficult periods in my life, I am acutely aware of my inexperience in helping, and I feel like anything I say could be perceived as trite or full of platitudes. I typically just try to listen as much as possible and, for example, ask the person about their support networks, where they could go for more professional, expert support – without seeking to offer any too tangible advice – as I'm acutely aware of my skill set and role in the conversation.

Jess is spot on with how she responds to that sense of helplessness, which is, in short, to not get caught up in overthinking your lack of experience; instead, simply listen and encourage the person toward the right support. You don't have to be the fixer or expert and it's not always about saying the right thing; it's about being there for someone.

TRY THIS …

This exercise will help you practise sitting with silence. Set an alarm for say ten minutes (longer if you can and want to). Sit in a comfortable position, with a sense of intention – this is not a relaxation exercise; it might be described as mindfulness or just call it sitting, breathing and noticing if that's more comfortable. Try to do this exercise with self-kindness; it's not about doing it right or wrong, it's just about doing it.

- Close your eyes and begin to feel your breath as you breathe in and then out. There is no need to breathe in any particular way.
- Where do you notice your breath? In your belly? Chest? Nostrils? Make wherever you notice the breath most naturally your anchor, the place you bring your attention back to when it wanders … and it will wander, because that is what our minds do!
- Now simply sit, notice and repeat.
- Each time your mind wanders, gently bring your attention back to your breath.
- Once you've completed the sitting, enjoy a moment of reflection. What happened? What feelings and thoughts came up for you? How do you feel now compared to before you started?
- Write down your reflections if that helps.

If you don't want to practise being silent alone, listen to an episode of Steve Chapman's 100-episode strong podcast *The Sound of Silence* (www.soundofsilence.org.uk) and join Steve and his guest for a sit in silence.

IT'S OKAY!

I love my conversations with Sulaiman Khan and his endorsement of "silence" is a great big fist-bump of okay which I'm grateful for. He explains:

It's okay to have silence in a conversation, yet often we want to shut out the silence with noise. Sometimes we just need to sit with our emotions, sit with the feelings and sit with the awkwardness and know that's okay. And when it comes to the conversations themselves it's okay to make mistakes, you're not always going to get everything right. For me it's always about progression over perfection.

Silence is a Gift

Yes, a pause, a period of silence, might feel uncomfortable at first, but when we reframe it as a gift and as a way to connect with someone and simply be there for them, everything changes, we *feel* different, more comfy, more compassionate. Remember the evidence for the deep-rooted human instinct and reward giving and gifting others? So, own the awkward pause, Own Your Awkward and help them own theirs, just by listening. The gift of silence says "No rush", "I'm here", "In your own time".

NOTEPADS TO ONE SIDE

My sister Susie has her own experience of mental ill-health, and her story illustrates the importance of noticing and asking if someone is okay:

I have watched other people live with poor mental health, but when I was struck with anxiety, panic attacks and paranoia, I began to really understand the impact it can have on our lives – not wanting to get on a train, socialize, talk to friends or family or become a burden to the people around me. In the past work had been my coping mechanism, my "go to" when my mental health was low, but this time work was the trigger for my poor mental health. For 12–18 months I'd experienced different challenges at work and done my best to remain professional and "park" my feelings in a box and carry on. What I couldn't see was the box getting full and beginning to overflow.

It was during a meeting that I hit a wall. I was asked how I was feeling, how was I really feeling? For the first time the notepads and agendas had been put to one side and someone was asking me how I felt. The smile I'm often known for disappeared and my body began to collapse. My shoulders fell and I cried more than I had for a long time as I began to tell them how I really felt. This was my awkward moment; I didn't know what reaction I was going to get and that was scary, but the two women in front of me showed me nothing but kindness and support. The conversation I had been trying to avoid was happening and it was okay,

> *I wasn't being judged, and I felt like someone was look-*
> *ing after me and cared about my mental health. These two*
> *women had noticed that something was wrong, and they*
> *helped me by starting the conversation that others hadn't.*
>
> Susie's story shows the importance of not only starting
> the conversation, but then holding the space for someone
> so that they can experience the great relief and release of
> letting go of the difficult feelings they have been carrying
> and trying to mask.

Embracing the Pause

When we embrace a deeper way of listening, we'll inevitably experience and notice more silences as a result, because some of them will come from you. When someone has shared some of what they are feeling, a natural pause will arise. You may want to respond and reply, make sure they feel okay, that they feel heard – after all that's an important part of demonstrating you are engaged and doing that listening job – but I encourage you to view the silence that follows as a gift to you this time. Utilize each pause to thoughtfully consider and craft your next response. No rushing required. Wiser responses are constructed as a result of embracing the pause.

Attention signals trust.

Listening creates trust.

Hearing nurtures trust.

Don't just listen, hear.

Supporting Our Intuition and Our Sixth SENSE

Being quiet, being silent ... both give our senses and intuition space to hone and fine-tune, to become stronger, more effective and of greater use to us. A pause, a few quiet seconds or even a minute and our senses become sharper, more tuned in and we become better placed to pick up other signals and signs, the less obvious, the unsaid, that can help us begin to build a picture of what is going on for someone. Silence can give our intuition greater space and capacity to work harder from and it can help us set ourselves up more confidently to ask the questions that help tease out a little more detail, some more of the story or situation, and often that helps uncover the real issue or challenge, the real response to "How are you?". It can help us pick up that we need to perhaps ask the more awkward question, in service to helping the person we want to support.

Using the Power of the Pause Tactically

Consider how you can use the awkward pause tactically (in the most caring of ways, of course) to gently elicit a response. Remember, if *you* don't speak and fill the silence, the other person likely will. So, in a way, silence helps keep the conversation going, without you having to keep it going and it helps it stay on the terms of the person you are talking to.

The journalist and documentary maker Louis Theroux is a master of using the power of the pause to keep a conversation going and help his interviewees to open up gradually. He 100% Owns His Awkward too. Holding silence is part of his toolkit and he accompanies it with a well-practised deadpan expression, serving to ensure he's not leading someone's response and the direction of the conversation too much through overly emoting, and he lets moments speak for themselves. Even if they are awkward. Watch his interviews and you'll see silence in action.

I use the power of the pause when I'm delivering mental health training. Sometimes I'll ask the group what they think about a film, an exercise or simply how they are feeling. I'll tactically use the power of the pause to generate responses because, guaranteed, if I don't speak or move the conversation on, someone in the group will respond and "save" me from the silence. I'll push it further, use another pause and more often than not someone else will again fill the silence, usually with another gem, insight or observation that will be incredibly useful to the group and that might not have been shared if I'd kept things moving. It's a natural human response to want to fill the silence, even if you are the one struggling to find the words or share your feelings. Embrace the tumbleweed moment and own it.

LORI'S "LOST" YEAR

Lori Zimmer is the author of *Art Hiding In New York*. We met at Miami Basel, an annual art fair. She sprang to mind for this book, as I had seen her fully owning her awkward, all the way across the pond in New York, where she lives, in tandem with me owning mine. Lori's story echoes so much of my own experience, not only the awkward, but also how such tumultuous and terrible times can bring gifts such as a much-needed pause and sometimes even a change of direction, stronger friendships and relationships and a better understanding of ourselves. It also serves to point out in her experience of grief that silence can sometimes feel uncaring if tied up in an awkward moment that is not owned. She told me:

An awkward pause was an opportunity for an awakening, a gift, a surprise ending to a difficult time.

My awkward pause came in the form of an entire year. It started when I donated my kidney to a friend, and kicked into high gear when my father died two weeks after my surgery. The altruistic high I was supposed to feel from saving someone's life after the pain subsided was instead taken over by intense grief, and the utterly empty feeling of unfairness. The flood of confusing emotions transformed my usually chipper, social butterfly self into a self-focused homebody, surprisingly, much to the chagrin of most of my network.

Before my "lost" year started at the end of 2018, my life was centred in the art world. Many of my friends and acquaintances were artists and art world people I'd helped in some way or another; writing articles about their work or shows, curating them into exhibitions, introducing them to other movers and shakers. It was a nonstop, often thankless job, but I thrived on making connections for other people, it gave me a sort of high. When I donated my kidney, a few sent flowers, but when my father died, most were silent (in fact, many I never heard from again). Those who did reach out had ulterior motives (can you give me so and so's number? Can you connect me with such and such magazine?) and if I'd accidentally mention my inability to help because I was paralysed by my overwhelming grief, I was met with deafening silence.

Despite the awkward responses I received that year (or lack thereof), I decided to go against my gut and remain open about my grief and depression. I saw it not just as a teachable moment for others (as we can all expect loved ones to die), but also as a selfish but necessary step for me, I needed to fully feel every painful pang in order to get through it. I'm not going to lie, for the most part, it really sucked. Losing "friends" after losing a dad (and a kidney) was something I didn't anticipate. But for every few acquaintances who decided they didn't have an interest in dealing with me when I wasn't my best, a good friend became a GREAT one.

As the months passed, the revelations came. I completely lost interest in writing articles and curating art shows, a career I'd dedicated ten years of my life building. I thought maybe I was just too depressed to organize something as social as an art show. But as the time passed, I realized I'd been unhappy in that world for a long time and that it was no longer serving me; only I never had the time to see it. The disappearance of that part of my network emphasized that maybe it just wasn't for me anymore.

Realizing what I no longer wanted set me on an important and incredible path. My depression and grief were becoming unbearable and started to unearth other mental issues I'd never dealt with. Because of my grief, I finally came to terms with seeing a therapist, something I'd been terrified of for years. Dedicating the time (and money) specifically toward my mental health was a major step that began to turn the gravity of my grief. Because I no longer wanted to make a living curating art shows (and had time on my hands), I enrolled in a creative writing class. My depression changed my day-to-day life, and I began enjoying working alone, away from the constant buzz I was used to. Without my social obligations, I had time to work on an art history writing project I'd been kicking around for years. Soon, I found myself surprisingly happily deep in the research, and my project blossomed into a full-on book. I sent it to a friend who I hoped would add her incredible illustrations, and she was just as excited as I was. We decided to keep going until we felt it was finished, with an idea to self-publish at the end. When it was done, I sent it to an agent friend to get her opinion. She loved it, signed us immediately, and quickly sold the manuscript to a leading publisher.

I thank the universe every day for that terrible year. It was both the worst and best thing to ever happen to me. My depression blew up my life completely, and in turn allowed me to shed the things that were weighing me down – people, jobs, habits, and raised up the positives in my life – the friends who stuck around, my relationship, my passion for writing that I didn't have time for before. I let my depression take over, I let it wash over me, and

I let it guide me to a new place, a place entirely and purposefully chosen by me. It may be a cliché of hitting rock bottom before climbing high, but I am left with a life I've chosen, friends who check in with each other openly and empathetically about mental health, a boyfriend I know will support me through thick and thin, and a career that leaves me fulfilled instead of depleted. Being awkward and open about my mental health led me to an open and honest life, on a messy, painful and rewarding path.

There are so many "That's Me" moments when I read Lori's story, the only part I'd challenge is when she says she went against her gut and continued to communicate openly about her grief and depression. I'd offer that perhaps, in fact, she was listening and responding to it and I for one am glad she did.

Just Pause

Pause to support your own health – physical, mental and emotional. Pause and make space internally to notice and slow down unhelpful chatter and externally to stop, make space, go a little slower if that is what you need, or faster if that's what's needed.

LISTENING SKILLS

Despite your best efforts, when you are in any kind of conversation, your mind will wander and you'll find it almost impossible to not drop, either frantically, thoughtfully, or both, into trying to work out how to respond. There's also the risk of concentrating so hard on listening well and not letting your mind wander that you become almost robot-like, on auto-response, which is equally awks! The task is listening to understand, listening to connect and listening to hear what is *really* being said. We can only begin to do that when we are committed to listening well, listening better and listening to truly hear. When we give someone our full attention, we want them to *feel* that attention and care, really feel it – and believe me they *will* feel it if it's authentically there, which, by the way, means they *will* feel it if it's not authentically there.

BEING PART OF EACH OTHER'S WELLBEING TOOLKIT

Poppy Jaman is CEO of City Mental Health Alliance and Founder of Rebalance; she also founded MHFA England. We met whilst trekking in Ecuador (for more on this, see page 165). You know you've made a friend for life when within days, hours even, you are sharing tents, snacks, stories and fears, and even the odd rock when there are no toilets for miles or hours, all whilst howling with laughter at something ridiculous in one moment and plotting to save the world in the next.

I appreciate the brutal honesty Poppy brings to a reflection about conversations she did and didn't have with her daughter and the importance of deep listening, truly hearing and creating the space, the pause, to enable that.

She also reminds us, as I shared at the beginning of this book, that sometimes we will have regrets and how important it is that we forgive ourselves when a conversation doesn't always go well because, let's be honest, we won't always get it right. She told me:

Learning to listen is a skill and it's something we need to build throughout life; it's not something we can become complacent about – a lesson that took me by surprise within my own family.

When my daughter stepped into her teenage years, she started expressing challenges at school, not with education but with social dynamics. At the time, I was working hard to build MHFA England, as well as renovating and literally building a new home for us. I was focused on giving my children choices by being financially healthy and, on this occasion, despite being an expert and "professional" listener, I missed the early warning signs. I did not listen to what my daughter was saying to me in a deep way.

I was grateful that I had parented my children to know that help-seeking behaviour is a skill and not a weakness. Clearly that had landed as my daughter sought help from the school counsellor. She tried to talk to me, but I wasn't fully engaged. I suggested she tried different ways to engage with her social circles, I offered solutions but I hadn't recognized that she was being excluded and experiencing micro-aggressions from her peers that were massively eroding her confidence. If I had paused, noticed and approached her with curiosity and not with a standard "mum" response, I would have stepped in with all my skills. I wonder now whether at a deeper level I found it hard to address the situation because it was too painful and I couldn't protect her or empower her; maybe on some level I saw this as my failure – this is what mental health stigma does, even to those of us that have been working in this space all our lives.

I'm grateful that my girl is independent and values herself enough to seek help. I'm regretful that she was riddled with guilt about accessing therapy without my knowledge. I think we underestimate how powerful our approval, support and judgement are to young teenagers. A few sessions into her school counselling and she found the energy to re-engage me, because she recognized that I am part of her wellbeing toolkit. Our relationship is crucial to both of our wellbeing. I am glad to say that we have an awesome relationship and she is thriving now. Her wisdom always floors me. She is my best teacher.

A 2015 survey by the Time To Talk campaign in the UK found that over 50% of parents had never had a conversation with their children about mental health, because they either didn't know how to or didn't think they needed to. The research estimates 1 in 10 children will experience a mental health problem and we know that getting help, as quickly as possible, will make all the difference. As we explored in Chapter 2, we *all* have mental health and that includes children and young people. Poppy reminds us of the role we play in teaching them that asking for help is a critical skill.

How to Listen So That You Can Hear

Samaritans is a UK-based charity that provides free emotional support to anyone in need, primarily through a volunteer-run telephone helpline. It was one of the first organizations we supported through Pjoys, after I met Ruth Sutherland, the outgoing CEO, and now Chair of Social adVentures in the UK, at an event we were both speaking at. I enthusiastically told her about the imminent launch of Pjoys and how we'd love to create a partnership with the charity. She replied, "It sounds wonderful Michelle, but right now we have to give our full attention to supporting our front-line services, such is the demand." That was that, decision made; Samaritans would be our first beneficiary, no campaign required.

This is the Samaritans Listening Model. It's simple and effective and it deserves to be shared. You can use it alongside the SENSE framework.

Open questions	Use questions that don't require a yes or no answer.	"How?" "What?" "Where?" "Who?" "Why?"
Summarize	A summary helps to show the person that you have listened and understood their circumstances and their feelings.	"What I'm hearing is …"

Reflect	Repeating back a word or phrase encourages the person to carry on and expand.	Them: "It's just that life just seems too much at the moment." You: "It seems too much?"
Clarify	The person may gloss over an important point. By exploring these areas further, we can help them clarify these points for themselves.	"Tell me more about that …"
Short words of encouragement	The person may need help to go on with their story.	"Yes, mmm, go on, it's okay."
React	Show you have understood by reacting verbally and non-verbally.	"It's brave of you to share how you are feeling."

Body Language

We have two ears, one mouth, providing a simple formula and ratio (even for the mathematically challenged like me) for listening versus talking. We communicate far more non-verbally (65%) as opposed to verbally (35%). So, considering your body language and actions as much as the words you speak is an essential part of communication.

- As the British businesswoman Sháá Wasmund MBE offers, "Listen with your ears *and* your eyes."
- Keep eye contact, but don't stare. If the person seems uncomfortable with eye contact, that's okay – look at their mouth, hands or maybe in the direction they are looking.
- Lean slightly forward to demonstrate your interest in what they are saying. If you can, avoid direct face-to-face sitting (yes, we are embracing the awkward, but let's avoid intensifying the awkward; it's not a game of chess). Try sitting at a comfortable angle, with no desk in between you if you're in an office.
- Be still (but not like a mannequin, because that would be beyond awkward). Just don't fidget or distract with any habits like biting your nails, winding your hair, jiggling your leg.
- Oh, and please put your phone away.

We can also pick up signals, signs and a deeper sense of someone's story and situation by tuning into their body language and actions. Closed body, head in hands, fidgeting, hunched shoulders, fast breathing, shallow breathing, shoulders tensed, facial expressions, tone of voice, sighing, pace of talking, lack of eye contact and more, tell us so much, when someone is maybe not yet saying very much at all.

TRY THIS …

Even with the best of intentions to listen fully and truly hear, we'll find our attention drifting elsewhere, for all

kinds of reasons – from daydreaming to solution-finding to unintentional distractions – because that is what the mind does. No need to beat yourself up about it. At the moment you realize you've drifted, try using a speedy Four-Step Reframe:

1. Stop and Notice (Oh heck, I've got distracted, etc.)
2. Acknowledge and Name (I feel embarrassment, guilt, I'm uncaring, etc.)
3. Move and Breathe (Gently shift your body and notice your breath in and out)
4. Transform and Reframe (Moving and breathing can help me hear better; it's okay, the mind wanders, I'm tuning back in)

WEEDING-OUT CONVERSATIONS

Stormie Mills and my husband Remi have a brotherly love and connection, and whilst he lives so far away from us, in Australia, with his wife Melissa, they have remained close ever since they first met, many moons ago, at a Graffiti Jam in Birmingham, England. You don't need to live close to someone to provide them with support. A successful artist, Stormie's work is often about communicating the isolation and loneliness he felt as a child, with his experience of homelessness shaping many of the stories his work tells. For me his characters sometimes feel sad, yet always tender, often with a sense of awkwardness and yet eternally hopeful – I connect with them. He encouraged and joined me for some gentle runs whilst he stayed with us during a trip to London, at a point in my life when I really needed to find a way to move my body but felt too awkward to do so on my own.

Stormie reflects that awkward conversations can sometimes shine a spotlight on the people you want to be around more and those who maybe you don't (see more about this in Chapter 9 when we explore Drains and Radiators):

I don't think it's as awks for me as it is for some other people to talk about my mental health. I think for an artist it is easier sometimes, although that doesn't always mean it is well received. Some people don't "get it" – those that think it's better that you deny not feeling good mentally, or they just don't want to know. So, for me it's only awkward when the person I'm talking to isn't on my wavelength. My wife Melissa and I check in with each other's mental health and wellbeing a lot and I have come to understand, that for me a real friend is someone who will listen when things need to be discussed. At this stage of my life, I don't want so many people around me who only have a surface understanding of me or the world, so sometimes those more "difficult conversations" are also good "weeding-out conversations".

The more we help others Own Their Awkward, by owning ours, the less likely our friends and families will fall through the gaps and out of our lives, due to being too afraid to embrace the awkward conversations in life.

THE CORNERSTONES OF AWKWARD CONVERSATIONS

Confidence

Now you know that silence is a gift, not something to be afraid of or fill immediately.

Capability

Use the Samaritans Listening Model to support your conversations and hear better.

Communication

We communicate far more non-verbally (65%) as opposed to verbally (35%). Use quiet moments to support your non-verbal communication.

Compassion

Attention signals trust.
Listening creates trust.
Hearing nurtures trust.

CHAPTER 7

The BRAVE Framework:
Asking for Help

"Challenges are gifts that force us to search for a new centre of gravity. Don't fight them. Just find a different way to stand."

Oprah Winfrey

After a brief interlude exploring the power of the pause, let's get going again and step into the second talking framework, BRAVE. Whilst it can feel awkward and overwhelming to start a conversation that's about supporting someone with *their* mental health, for many of us it can be even more challenging and awkward to talk about *our own* mental health, especially if we are experiencing issues with it.

SELF-CARE OR SELF-INDULGENT?

Years of stigma, shame and embarrassment, as well as simply not always recognizing or being familiar with the signs and symptoms of mental ill-health, mean we delay getting support, we pretend life is okay and we avoid asking for help for fear of how others will respond and view us. We stay quiet. I think it's fair to say that many of us are also incredibly hard on ourselves, with "self-love" and "self-care" being viewed as words and behaviours that are all too often tarnished with the "self-indulgent" brush. Guilty as charged ... until now.

With zero apologies, the final chapters of this book are dedicated to self-care, because at the very least, we should be placing *equal* importance on our own mental health and that of others, but let me push you a little further, what if we put understanding and looking after our own mental health first, as our priority? I put it to you that we'll be better placed to help others; with our confidence wobbling less, we'll have a greater capability and capacity to use the SENSE framework to support those who need us and start a conversation. Our communication will be clearer, calmer and more consistent, and we'll have an abundance of compassion as a result. Case closed.

That Oxygen Mask Analogy

The oxygen mask analogy has become more widely used recently, and for good reason, it works ... When you're on a plane the safety briefing says in an emergency place your own oxygen mask on before you begin to help others on with theirs.

The simple reason being, you are better placed to look after others when you are in the best possible place yourself.

And there's another reason for putting your own self-care first. Because as well as sometimes being awkward, supporting people with poor mental health can be hard, emotionally draining, mentally taxing and energy zapping and if we are trying to help others when our own mental health is declining, we're potentially risking the quality of the support we're offering others. You can't drink from an empty cup (and offering someone a drink from your empty cup isn't terribly useful either). Use what follows to replenish your reserves and if you can't find it in you to be kind to yourself and look after you for *you*, then at least do it so you can be a better support for *others*.

There's another bonus – you can add the self-care information and strategies you learn to your talking toolkit/handbag and share them with others. View it as useful content for awkward conversations and offering help.

The Vicious Cult of "I'm fine"

"How are you?"

"Fine, how are you?"

"I'm fine."

Sound familiar? The standard greeting of absolute nothingness. On page 55 we saw the cost of presenteeism, when employees go to work, but are not as productive as they might usually be due to undisclosed issues, including stress, not feeling secure at work or in their role, bullying, mental ill-health and more. Beyond the workplace, it's even more difficult to assess and estimate the impact of people going about their lives with the weight of undiagnosed, undisclosed and unsupported mental ill-health impacting their ability to cope with and enjoy a fulfilling life. From parents and carers, to the unemployed and self-employed, to students, retirees and children, the impact of not talking about our mental health is huge, for the individual and beyond, in terms of all the other areas their poor health reaches, influences and has an impact on. The vicious cult of "I'm fine" at its very worst.

I was a member of the "I'm fine" cult and, hey, it's still hard not to say it; it's so ingrained in my day-to-day language. I try to avoid it, though, and do my best to answer the question "How are you?" honestly. Whilst sometimes taking people by surprise, an honest response usually feels good and I've found it can set up a conversation better and more interestingly than the bog standard, utterly boring exchange of "I'm fine", even if I'm giving the more awkward and honest response that I'm not or haven't been feeling great.

I've come to accept that understanding my mental health and ill-health will likely be a lifelong journey, as my own story, experience and Life Footprint all continue to grow and play out over time, in ways that I can hope, dream and plan for but not in any way guarantee or know for sure, because hopes and dreams are not facts. Fact.

Stuck in the Bottom-Right Quadrant

Remember the Mental Health Continuum (see page 29) and how being stuck in that bottom right-hand quadrant is where the problems can escalate? It's where we're most likely to be silently struggling, confused about what we are experiencing, afraid to say it aloud, searching for the words to describe how and what we are feeling, or perhaps burying our difficulties so deep that we have become almost oblivious to them ourselves; denying our truth, we keep on keeping on. This is not the way to live our lives and it doesn't have to be so.

THE BRAVE TALKING FRAMEWORK

Be aware – Of how you are feeling and coping with life.
Remember – You are not alone.
Ask for help – From someone you trust
Value yourself – You are not a burden.
Explore what helps – We are all different.

I developed the BRAVE framework to help people take those first steps to asking for help. So why BRAVE? The origins of the word "courage" come from the Old French *corage*, and *cuer* and ultimately from the Latin *cor*, all meaning "heart". Bravery is the ability to face danger or pain. It is about activating the mental and moral strength to face that danger and pain. Bravery takes courage in the mind, body, spirit *and* heart. Especially so when we are the ones asking for help. Especially when it feels awkward. But where to start?

Asking for help can be hard and to be able to ask for help, we need to acknowledge that we need it in the first place. Even harder than that is acknowledging that we deserve it, not just need it. We can be so compassionless for ourselves. BRAVE helps you *arrive* at the point of asking for help, as well as helping you stay there. It's as much about the conversation you have with yourself as it is others, and often there's more awkward to overcome before either of those conversations can even start. Feeling daunted? No need to be; you are here, this is the work. We have to keep being BRAVE when it comes to self-care and talking about our mental health and each letter and prompt is an ongoing reminder and ammunition for fighting off the advances of The Dirty Duo and their armies.

B for Be aware
... Of how you are feeling and coping with life.
- Make regular time to check in with yourself honestly.
- How are your confidence levels? How are you feeling about yourself? Your life?
- Use the Mental Health Continuum (see Chapter 2) and The Stress Dispenser and Exhaustion Funnel (see Chapter 8) to check in with your mood and stress levels.
- Notice how you are reacting, responding and behaving. Does it feel okay, good or helpful? Or is it difficult, unhelpful or painful even?
- How honest are you being with yourself about any of the above?

Ask yourself these questions with kindness, like you would if you were asking somebody else how they are doing. Be your own friend here and, as best you can, be honest with yourself. Maybe you can ask someone you trust how *they* think you are doing. Sometimes others can see the issues before we can ourselves.

R for Remember
... You are not alone.

- We all have mental health, and we'll all experience the ups and downs in life. You're not alone.
- Thoughts are not facts, and you are not your thoughts.
- It's more common to experience poor mental health than perhaps you know.
- You might not have the words to describe or understand what you are experiencing. That's okay, it's understandable. When you begin to talk, the words will come.
- What would you say to a friend or family member experiencing similar kinds of thoughts?

Experiencing poor mental health can feel incredibly lonely and isolating and it's when those unhelpful thoughts can escalate. Finding ways to remind ourselves that having mental health issues is common and that no one should be alone with those thoughts is a good reminder and step toward asking for help.

A for Ask for help
... From someone you trust.

- Who do you know that is a good listener? Who can you talk easily to? Who do you trust?
  It might be family, friends, a co-worker, a teacher, perhaps a medical professional like your doctor or nurse.
- If you can't think of someone specific, calling, emailing, or texting a helpline or service can be a good first step (see the Useful Resources section on page 265). Talking anonymously could be good.

- Can you pinpoint what is stopping you from asking for help? Do you have evidence? Try the Four Steps To Owning Your Awkward exercise (see page 80) to help reframe any unhelpful thoughts.
- Opening up about your feelings might be hard, but it's so worth trying.

Sometimes when you reach out for help, the person you talk to may not react the way you hoped or give you the support you have asked for, which can feel difficult. If that happens, remember that their reaction is about them, not you. We are all different and we won't all react or respond in the same way. Try not to be discouraged. Remember, there are so many people who will want to help you.

V for Value Yourself
... You are not a burden.

- You are not a burden. You have so much to offer.
- You don't have to be alone in this. People care and want to help you.
- You deserve to have support and you'll start to feel better when you get the right support.
- We often find it most difficult to be kind to ourselves. It might take practice, but give it a go.
- Value yourself in the same way you value the people you care about.

Sometimes you have to take a deep breath and just believe the above points, even when you can't see them or feel them. Just know that you *are* loved and valued.

E for Explore What Helps
... We are all different.

- Help for mental ill-health looks like different things to different people.
- There's not necessarily a right or wrong; it's about finding what works for you.
- Much of mental health treatment and support is about chemistry and relationships. It might take time to find the right professional relationship for you. It's okay if the first one doesn't work, but it doesn't mean that none will. The same goes for taking medication.
- There are so many routes to recovery and so much of it is about treating the person, not the illness. You are a beautiful, unique human being after all.
- Patience and perseverance are important. Give it time.

There really are so many ways of supporting mental ill-health, and it can take time to find what's best for you for all kinds of understandable, yet also frustrating, reasons. As much as you can, try keeping an open mind to the various options available and offered to you and keep going.

A CONVERSATION WITH MYSELF

Jo Davey, a Talent Director I work with, demonstrates through her own story of mental illness how the step before the BRAVE act of asking for help is often the one where we must have that awkward conversation with ourselves. She told me:

I think the most awkward conversation was the one I had to have with myself when I woke up one morning, after the most gruelling of six-month pitches, with a swollen face and the recognition that I had completely burnt out and was broken mentally and physically. I had to say to myself "enough is enough, you cannot outrun this, you need to stop – you are a mum and a human and there is another way."

My husband, my mum, my co-workers, my friends had been saying this to me for months (probably years), but more acutely in the last six months. They didn't understand why I continued to push myself beyond all reasonable expectations to deliver for others – with no care for what it was doing to myself. The anxiety I had been experiencing over the last six months was chronic, so bad that I remember sitting in a café with my family, on a rare Saturday that I wasn't working, with so much adrenaline in my body that I was shaking. I remember feeling completely trapped and hopeless.

The night I realized that enough really was enough, I woke up at 3am and Googled, "How to commit suicide". I remember the time of night, where I was and exactly how I felt. I remember vividly I just wanted the feelings in my brain to stop, I felt terribly alone and truly felt at that moment that the world would be better off without me.

I scared myself and the next day I got an emergency appointment with my doctor, went back on antidepressants and got referred to a counsellor. I left my job and began the gruelling six months to get myself back to health. It could have been different for me – suicide is a heart attack of the brain and in that moment of darkness I had just enough strength to hold on and wait for the doctor's surgery to open to get help. Others won't be that lucky.

One in four people experience suicidal thoughts – they are more common than we might think or expect. Talking about these feelings can help prevent them from escalating. If you are experiencing these kinds of thoughts, please talk to someone and use the Useful Resources on page 265.

TRY THIS …

Think about what barriers and blockers might be stopping you from asking for help? The things you think might be a negative consequence? How you'll be viewed (judged)? How it makes you feel? Worry? (Say after me: "Worry is manufactured and a waste of time Michelle.")

If it helps, begin by thinking about examples that aren't specifically about mental health – the other things in life that you find hard to ask for help with – perhaps chores at home, support for family members, workload, finding time to look after yourself. What's preventing you from asking for support? Could you use one of these challenges to practise asking for help? Then graduate your thinking and asking to your mental health and wellbeing.

Note down something you find difficult to ask for help. Now note all the different thoughts and barriers using these prompts. Here's a helping hand to get you started:

When asking for help with your workload you might be thinking:

"What if my co-workers think I can't cope."

"I might lose my job."

"They might think I'm incompetent."

"It might mean I don't get a promotion."

"I'm embarrassed to say I can't cope."

- What if ...
- I might ...
- They might ...
- It might ...
- I can't ...
- I haven't ...
- It's impossible ...
- I am ...
- I'm not ...

Now take each of your barriers and blockers and use the Four Steps To Owning Your Awkward to see how you can think about the situation differently, flip it, Transform and Reframe.

1. Stop and Notice
2. Acknowledge and Name
3. Move and Breathe
4. Transform and Reframe

Taking the example used above you might reframe as:

"I might get even better at my job because I asked for space/help."

"They might feel a good sense of teamwork because I asked for help."

"It might benefit me in all the right ways to ask for support."

"I am a valued member of the team and I also value myself."

"I am human, it's okay to ask for help."

- What if ...
- I might ...
- They might ...
- It might ...
- I can't ...
- I haven't ...
- It's impossible ...
- I am ...
- I'm not ...

By trying this exercise, you are creating space and permission to get out of the chitter-chatter in your head and look at and approach the situation differently. It might not work every time, but how great if it works some of the time?

MY TURN TO BE BRAVE

In the second half of 2019, from a place of recovery, I was racing, perhaps faster and faster, as is my way when some good, positive momentum in life and work gets going. We had taken Pjoys to London Fashion Week invited by Caroline Rush, CEO of the British Fashion Council, as part of their Positive Fashion showcase – an intense, but overwhelmingly proud and prestigious experience. We were about to launch exclusively in Fenwick of Bond Street, London, where we had a window display to create, and two events instore to plan for our launch there on World Mental Health Day and, of course, there was the pushing and refining of our direct sales and communications through our own Pjoys platform.

On top of that, my speaking requests were growing, as were bookings for my corporate training sessions. I was also continuing with my commitments to Livity, supporting the business side of Remi's work and Lili was working toward her GCSE mock examinations – oh and I'd started on the physical training for a trek in Ecuador, more of which shortly. Uh oh! It was feeling particularly hard to "not work too hard" and embrace "slowly but joyfully", the mantras and promises made to myself after my burnout. I noticed my mood beginning to fluctuate.

Thoughts of Death

At the start of one week, I felt highly anxious, and the familiar storm cloud had moved right back above my head and didn't seem to be shifting. The Dirty Duo – depression and anxiety – were back in town, sitting menacingly on each shoulder, cawing like crows. Birds are brilliant! I love them increasingly as I get older; I even have a bird book to identify the lesser-spotted bird species of South London, as I sit looking out at my garden as mindfully as I can, but I find crows have an air of menacing unfriendliness about them. The Royal Society for the Protection of Birds (RSPB) describe crows as "one of the cleverest, most adaptable birds, often quite fearless, although wary of man. They are solitary, usually found alone, or in pairs. They will come into gardens for food and although often cautious initially, they soon learn when it is safe, and will return repeatedly to take advantage of whatever is on offer." Oh, hi, The Dirty Duo. Hello mental ill-health.

As well as the usual unwelcome feelings The Dirty Duo bring, this time there was something else lurking as well, something that felt deeply uncomfortable and a bit scary. What to do? Ask for help! That was the rallying cry I was sharing by this time with others day in and day out, and so it was time to take my own advice. "Don't sit with this on your own Michelle," I reminded myself, even though I really didn't want to say out loud what I was experiencing; in fact, once again I found myself searching for the words and this time it felt like a different, more sinister kind of uncomfortable.

I explained to Rumina, my therapist, that I was experiencing a real rollercoaster with my moods, but that I'd also found myself thinking about death an awful lot, like almost all the time. Saying it out loud made me cry. I didn't *feel* like it was suicidal thinking, but thoughts of death, whether it be mine, Remi's or Lili's were taking up far too much of my mind, including some uncomfortable impulses, which was the aspect really frightening me, and with the Dirty Duo back flip-flopping my mood, it all felt unpleasant. It should be noted, I was also experiencing brilliant days in-between these difficult ones. Our mental health can be complex!

When you have experienced periods of such difficult mental illness, you can be quite afraid of it happening again. I was terrified of falling into a similar place to the one I'd experienced in 2016/17. Rumina was, as ever, so great, non-judgemental, a brilliant and thoughtful listener and she agreed that maybe there was something more ongoing, something that had possibly been chugging along in the background that had not been specifically identified during my big burnout moment. She referred me to a psychiatrist she worked with and just a few weeks later I was sat in The Priory Hospital, with Dr Az Hakeem, who gave me two of the most helpful words in my mental health journey yet: Emotional Dysregulation.

Emotional Dysregulation (ED), also called "emotional hyper-activity", means that you are more emotionally responsive than an average person. Your emotions will be triggered more quickly and will tend to be on a bigger scale. Of course, most information about ED focuses on the ways it makes life challenging, more angry, tearful, sad, anxious or fearful, but you can also be more deeply touched by things like art and music than others, and be able to experience profound joy. You might find that you also have a talent for showing empathy.

Like most psychological conditions, there is no exact answer for why someone might have ED. It varies by the individual and tends to be a mix of biological and environmental factors. Temperament, childhood trauma, as well as recent trauma, can also cause ED. Trauma affects the brain, leaving it less able to manage stress.

Az's view was that I wasn't fitting neatly into one category of mood dysregulation (as we're learning, mental illness and humans can be complex!). He did, though, have a good sense of me and prescribed a medication to help manage the fluctuating emotions. I'd not felt quite ready for medication previously, but having put myself front and centre of the topic of mental illness over the last three years, I had reached a point where I felt open to trying medication, certainly for this issue and how it was impacting me, as long as it was alongside other treatments, supports and daily disciplines to look after my mental health.

I've heard many people talk about medication in a way that has evolved my view of it, but particularly recall listening to the actor Kristen Bell talk to her husband Dax Shepard on his Podcast, *The Armchair Expert*, about taking daily medication. The way she spoke about it, as part of her "normal" day-to-day and life in general was one of the things that helped me turn a corner in terms of how I felt about adding medication into the mix of treatment to help manage my mental health. She said, "I take a medication that helps balance me and I've become habitual about doing the things that make me feel good." Simple and honest stigma smashing at its best.

The medication worked for me, it helped, it's still helping, and it's still currently part of my self-care toolkit and plan. Part, not all.

Organizing Recovery Around Meaning and Purpose

I love delivering MHFA and the other mental health training sessions that I've designed for clients. I often feel at my most purposeful and comfortable when I'm taking people through a training session, giving them frameworks and that all important sense of confidence and capability. Plus, it's something I feel confident in delivering. Like most of us, I find it difficult to say that I'm any good at doing "stuff", but you know what? I *am* good at delivering mental health training and it was an invaluable part of my recovery and rebuilding my self-esteem.

In MHFA training, just toward the end of the final session, we show a short clip of a lecture given by Dr Pat Deegan. It makes me tingle every time I show it and, more often than not, I shed a tear. There are two things that stand out in Pat's lecture. The first is the idea of "Survivors Mission" – going on to do positive and transformative work related to the very trauma and illness one has experienced, and the second being that you can't organize a recovery from mental illness around a vacuum of "nothing"; you need to organize recovery around something that provides a sense of meaning and purpose alongside a sense of moving forward. Pjoys, mental health training and this book are clearly my own Survivors Mission, and the purpose and meaning that I built my own recovery around.

And all of *that* comes from taking ownership of that awkward comment and learning how to talk more freely and honestly about mental health.

And *that* came from finally being BRAVE enough to ask for, and crucially, accept help.

AN INVITATION I COULDN'T REFUSE (EVEN THOUGH I WANTED TO)

Halfway through 2019 I was connected to someone at HSBC to talk about an initiative they were leading to raise awareness and money for mental health charities and the wider topic itself. I had been impressed to learn about the bank's commitment to supporting good mental health and conversations about it.

Scott Pendrey, an Englishman living in San Francisco, was the HSBC contact and in our first conversation we formed a connection talking about mental ill-health – because that's what happens when you live in a world where you are Owning Your Awkward! Scott told me about an ambition he had to bring together 100 of his HSBC co-workers from around the globe and trek as one group to help start more conversations about mental health, both on the trip and beyond. He was looking for two or three ambassadors to join the trek, led by Charity Challenge. After some more sharing of stories and ambitions, he asked me if I'd join the seven-day, high-altitude volcano trek across the Andes in Ecuador, as one of the ambassadors. Wow, what an opportunity to do something so aligned to my own personal and professional mission. How could I say no?

"No"

"No, Scott. I'd love to, I'd be honoured, but no, I'm sorry, I'm afraid I can't. I won't be able to. You see, I'm just not fit enough and I have some pretty big challenges with exercise at the moment." I went on to explain that due to years of repeated abdominal medical procedures and complications, plus the mental illness that had impacted my physical health, I was weak, unfit and had developed an emotional anxiety response that was triggered every time I attempted any exercise, from running outdoors to being on the yoga mat indoors, from the real life gym to online programmes. I'd tried lots of times, but The Dirty Duo would rear their ugly heads every time I attempted to re-engage with exercise. As I quickly became out of breath or felt physically weak, the negative and unhelpful unkind chatter and squawking from them would commence – "You're so weak, you're so unfit, you're so old and you've left this fitness lark far too long to be able to improve now" and on it would go, increasing in intensity just at the same moment that my heart rate was rising. I'd get a lump in my throat and my eyes would sting, making it all the harder to breathe and it would mount and intensify until I had no capacity to continue; often I would silently weep, sometimes I'd loudly and breathlessly blub. I just felt so ashamed of my physical weakness, my lack of strength and any semblance of fitness or capacity for physical endurance.

"Yes"

Talking it through with Scott, I could see that here was yet another very live and present self-stigmatizing train of thought I was living with. I asked a few more questions about the trip and fitness requirements and then I heard myself saying, "Well if it's not until March maybe this is the kind of goal I need to overcome my fitness challenges. Okay Scott, if you think I can do it, then yes, I'm in." I hung up and thought to myself, "What the hell have I done?"

I Asked for Help

Alexandra McMillan is *my* Personal Trainer – even now it sounds strange writing those words. I brought all my honesty to that first session with Alex and she listened, without judgement, and spent time understanding me, my fears, my challenges and we then got to work on getting me physically and mentally fit for the trek.

And I did it. In March 2020, just as this emerging virus called Covid-19 seemed to be a bit of a growing issue, 100 of us met in Ecuador and walked, talked, cried, puffed, huffed and hugged and helped each other every step of the way to Mount Cotopaxi, and then we whooped and cheered and celebrated and reflected on just how many conversations we'd had about mental health and wellbeing and how many physical and metaphorical footsteps we had taken to get there. One moment I'd be crying as the incline NEVER ENDED and I felt I had nothing left in me, always with someone by my side, helping me on, step by step; the next we'd arrive on the flat (THANK YOU MOTHER NATURE), stop for a break and I'd deliver a mental health session, that every single time would connect with someone in the group and kickstart a beautiful conversation, for the next agonizing climb. People offered help and they asked for help across the seven days, across the group. Culture changing, stigma-smashing Superstars.

THE CORNERSTONES OF AWKWARD CONVERSATIONS

Confidence

Self-care gives space and support for confidence to grow.

Capability

You have the BRAVE framework. You might need to start with having an awkward conversation with yourself, to help you ask for help from others.

Communication

You are better placed to look after others when you are in the best possible place yourself. Remind yourself, tell others. It's an important message.

Compassion

The compassion starts with you. Self-care is not self-indulgent, it's smart. Recovery needs to be organized around purpose and mission, not a great big gap of nothingness.

CHAPTER 8

Wellbeing and Being Well

"We need to accept that we won't always make the right decisions, that we'll screw up royally sometimes – understanding that failure is not the opposite of success, it's part of success."

Arianna Huffington

Wellbeing is about feeling good and functioning well. It's the state of being comfortable, healthy and happy, and can be measured by how someone is thinking and feeling in terms of their life satisfaction, positive emotions, and whether their life is feeling meaningful alongside more basic human needs and rights such as food, health, education, safety, etc. Poor wellbeing can lead to poor mental health and poor mental health can contribute to poor wellbeing. Many research studies have shown that when we have good wellbeing, we live longer, we are happier, we are healthier (physically and mentally) and, overall, we seem to do better, both individually and collectively.

Wellbeing takes work and annoyingly there's not an exact formula or recipe for achieving it. There are, though, some key elements and ingredients that I'll share with you in the remaining chapters. But before we get into it, how are you? It's good to ask, right?

IT'S A WIN, WIN

I hope that by this point of the book your confidence has grown alongside your understanding of mental health and that you are thinking about embracing the power of sharing stories to help create "That's Me" moments of connection for others. I hope your capability is feeling bolstered, that you are Owning Your Awkward and using the SENSE framework to offer help to others and ready to use the BRAVE framework to ask for help as and when you need it. I hope you are appreciating the power of the pause and celebrating silence along the way – communication at its finest. You might be doing all of this joyfully, occasionally painfully, and most likely still a little AWKWARDLY; just know it's a proverbial "journey" and that we'll all go at different speeds, because there are different levels of awkward that we are now owning with a turbo-charged sense of compassion!

Now to explore the magic to the logic that weaves together all of what has gone before in this book and multiply its impact. It's that ever-so-slightly uncomfortable word that I whispered at the start of the previous chapter – go on, you can do it, say it out loud with me ... self-care.

Remember the oxygen mask analogy? When we take care of ourselves, we have more to give others. It's a win, win.

STRESSED?

"Stress" can sometimes be an easier way into the conversation about mental health than the words "mental health", and we want to find as many accessible shortcuts into the subject as possible, don't we? For many, "stress" is the more acceptable area of mental health language and definitions; it can be easier to talk about than mental ill-health and is seemingly easier to identify, even though most of the signs and symptoms fall into the same categories of diagnosable mental illnesses. There are differences, though, and certainly from my own experience being aware of and checking in with my own stress levels is a good starting point for regularly assessing my own mental health and wellbeing.

Stress was a major contributor to my burnout in 2016 and it's one of the expressions of the Fight, Flight, Freeze survival mechanism that we looked at in Chapter 3. A threatening situation will trigger a stress response in us, preparing us to physically confront or flee possible danger (remember that bear?). As we and the world around us have evolved, the stress response can also be triggered by everyday tense situations, such as dealing with an unreasonable co-worker, managing a heavy workload, juggling parenting, family and work, relationship issues, bad traffic, financial problems, to name just a few! Although these situations are stressful, our bodies are often shaking and serving up a cocktail of hormones that is far from good for our wellbeing and potentially disproportionate to the actual threat those stressful situations are presenting.

There are two types of stress to be aware of:

1. **Acute stress:** Prepares us for Fight or Flight, and is generally short-term.
2. **Chronic stress:** This is long-term and the main cause of stress-related health problems.

Stress can cause chemical changes in the body that, if left unchecked, can adversely affect both our mental and physical health, with high levels of stress contributing to health issues as diverse as depression, insomnia, heart disease, skin disorders and headaches. So, when you stop and think about it, understanding and managing stress is vital for our wellbeing, and for being well.

A note of caution: As you read this chapter, you might identify elements of your own stress that would benefit from support. If you do, this could be the time to use the BRAVE framework to talk about how you are feeling.

BREAKING POINT

Mervyn Lynn is a much-loved and respected consultant in the music industry. He is also Chair of The London Football Association's Inclusion Advisory Group. Whilst Vice President of Strategic Partnerships at the music giant, Sony Music Entertainment, he was one of the first people in the music industry to take a leadership role and do something about the lack of diversity in the sector (a mental health issue in its own right) and together, through my business Livity and Sony Music Entertainment, we created Music4Good. Merv shared with me an example of when the stress of work became so chronic it actually *scared* him into self-care – not the most joyful way to embrace the idea of taking care of ourselves. Why do we let ourselves get to breaking point before we ask for help or start looking after our mental health and wellbeing in the way we deserve? He told me:

I was working at Motown Records in the UK and looking after the Lionel Richie comeback album. I was spending an unrelenting amount of time between London and LA and calls would be required both early morning and late into the evening, due to the various time zones we were all working in. A week before the UK visit and album launch, for lots of different reasons, the trip and gig at the Hammersmith Odeon were cancelled. It was a massive blow and my stress levels were through the roof as I started to think about everything that needed to be done now the plan had changed so dramatically. After the worst of days and yet another late night at the office, I walked to my car, the weight of the world on my shoulders. As I walked past a building that had spotlights shining up and out from it, suddenly all I could see out of my left eye was a bright light – it was piercing, completely blinding me. It was probably for no more than a minute, but scary, nonetheless. My sight recovered and I got myself home.

Later that night the same thing happened again – the bright, blinding light. I couldn't even see my finger when I held it up in front of me. The following morning, I went to the opticians and was sent to Moorfields Eye Hospital, in London, and had what seemed like every test under the sun. Still no problem to be found. Eventually, I was diagnosed with having experienced a migraine, brought on due to immense stress. I was taken aback at how I could be impacted so physically by the stress of work and that day I vowed never to take work home, either literally or emotionally, again. Reflecting and realizing there was nothing I could do to change the fact that Lionel wouldn't be coming to the UK helped me put work into perspective, let it go and look after my own mental health better as a result.

Merv's story highlights how the physical response to stress often shows up more loudly and urgently than the mental and emotional; they are all so inextricably linked. It's those signs and signals again, communicating so much. And look how Merv reframed the situation to help himself. Accepting he couldn't do anything to change the situation allowed him to let it go.

THE STRESS DISPENSER

I'm going to share with you a tool that will help you become better equipped to understand and manage your stress, and once you understand how to use it for yourself, you can also use it to support others. It's based on a model originally developed by Professor Alison Brabban and Dr Douglas Turkington in 2002 and has been used by many organizations around the world, including MHFA England. It's been presented as stress buckets, funnels, containers and more. So, I now bring you my own zingy version of this valuable model that I've witnessed being useful time and time again. I call it The Stress Dispenser.

Vulnerability

Picture a lemonade or fruit punch dispenser. They come in all different sizes – some huge, big enough for catering at large events, some smaller, better for a BBQ perhaps, and very occasionally that embarrassing online purchase you make, thinking something is a "regular" size, but in fact it's a tiny dispenser for a doll's house – how awkward.

These dispensers can contain all kinds of delicious drinks – traditional lemonade, a fruit punch, perhaps with a splash of alcohol. Often they include chunks of fruit, juices, water or other drinks and perhaps even some herbs to add flavour. Getting the right combination of ingredients to achieve a perfect and palatable mix takes care and attention. Get the amounts wrong and it doesn't taste so good ...

Imagine that the dispenser represents the receptacle that receives, holds and releases stress, and the size of the dispenser represents the size of an individual's vulnerability and how much stress they are able to "hold" at any one time. Remember, this can vary a great deal, depending on all the things that make you YOU. The amount of stress we can take on and manage varies from person to person and some of us are more vulnerable to feeling the impact than others.

Managing Stress

Day to day, week to week, year to year, stress flows into and through our lives. Remember how I had "one of those years" in 2016 that led to my mental ill-health? Even though not everything in that year was bad, even the joyful things like my daughter starting a new school and Remi's career soaring could be described as additional stressors. Let's not demonize stress, though – it can motivate us, drive us, keep us safe, help us get somewhere on time, deliver to a deadline, help us pay attention more acutely, etc. What potentially creates problems is the cumulative impact of stress, and *how* we deal with it (or not) and that's where The Stress Dispenser becomes useful.

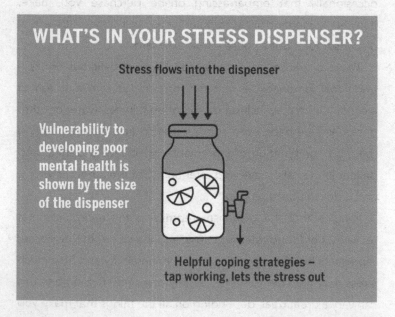

Like lemonade, stress flows (or pours) into the top of the dispenser

When we are managing stress well, everything is in working order and we're taking on and then releasing our stress just fine. We're using helpful coping and stress-releasing strategies, like moving regularly, talking, asking for help and support when we need it, as well as resting and getting a good night's sleep, etc. Picture that lovely cold lemonade being dispensed into your glass, taking a deep breath and relaxing as you take a sip.

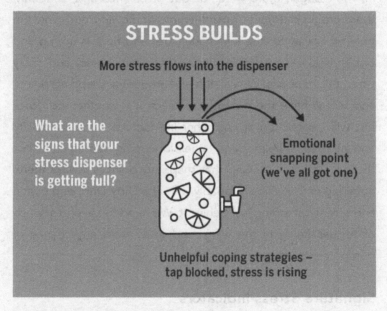

Stress builds up and the tap is jammed

Now imagine stress beginning to build up – let's say a few more big chunky lemons have been plonked into the dispenser, making the lemonade levels rise. As our dispenser begins to fill up, we may find ourselves turning more easily toward unhelpful coping strategies, like working longer and harder, eating food that is less nourishing, moving less, talking less, resting and recovering less. Another couple of lemons drop in and the lemonade levels are rising and now not tasting so good – they are out of balance, the dispenser is full to the brim and the dispensing tap is filling up with lemon pulp and getting jammed.

So, when stress increases we lose our steady flow, our tap might even get completely blocked. More chunks of lemon drop in, more sugar, more water, all out of balance and, suddenly, there are no delicious cups of lemonade flowing out. Now the only other way for the lemonade (stress) to flow, is up, up and out, eventually overflowing. It can get pretty messy and sticky when this happens. We call this an "emotional snapping point" and we *all* have the potential to reach it – whether we do or not will depend on all the other life factors, our vulnerability and our use of helpful and unhelpful coping strategies ... but the potential of reaching that snapping point is always there, hovering in the wings, probably with The Dirty Duo, depression and anxiety, standing just behind it. We need to keep this bunch of rogues firmly in the wings and away from any chance of getting centre stage.

Signature Stress Indicators

We all have our own signature stress indicators – the things that you (and often those around you) notice change or emerge when stress levels are rising. They often match or are influenced by unhelpful coping strategies. Mine include working longer, working harder, becoming snappy and distracted, feeling easily criticized, unhelpful chitter-chatter in my head, worrying about finances, craving comfort carbs, more frequent migraines, and I'm sure my family could tell you MORE signs than I can! Understanding what our own signature stress indicators look and feel like can be useful and aid us in making appropriate shifts and changes to our helpful and unhelpful coping strategies, and manage rising levels of stress. As we notice the indicators in ourselves, we can use them to be BRAVE and ask for help.

As well as using it for yourself, you can try The Stress Dispenser as a tool to talk to someone about their stress levels. With care and compassion, you can use it as a starting point for a conversation with the SENSE framework. Remember, though, it doesn't replace professional diagnosis and support.

TRY THIS …

Make a note of what stress is flowing into your Stress Dispenser now, keeping in mind that not all stress is bad.

- List the different things that are going on in your life? What do you notice about this list?
- List your *helpful* coping strategies for releasing stress?
- Note down the *unhelpful* coping strategies that you sometimes find yourself using to cope with stress? How does this list compare to the helpful coping strategies list? What triggers these unhelpful coping strategies? What could you do differently? What changes could you make and what help do you need to make them happen?

- Now identify your signature stress indicators. What are the signs and signals that you are aware of when your stress is rising and it's feeling difficult to cope? What do they look and feel like to you and to others? Which are the obvious ones, and which are the less obvious ones? Include those you're really not proud of (but go easy on yourself – it's just a list).
- With all of this information, now consider how you can weave moments of reflection into your life to check in on your stress and how you are managing it. Put time in your diary, a note on your mirror, a reminder in your phone to take a moment to check in on your Stress Dispenser.

BEING KIND TO YOURSELF

We run along in life, often racing, unaware of things beginning to pile on top of one another, with more and more "lemons" dropping into our Stress Dispenser, filling it up more quickly, putting a greater strain on the tap. There's not enough time (we tell ourselves) to use our helpful coping strategies, with more of the unhelpful coping strategies becoming part of our normal day-to-day living.

When you take a moment to review life and what's going on for you, it's a moment of self-care. You might be surprised and taken aback at just how many plates you are spinning and how some of those plates are bigger and take more of your attention and energy than others. So, when you stop, be gentle with yourself, notice what's going on, take a moment to think about what you could do more of or less of to manage your "lemonade" levels. This is where the M-Plan comes into play in the next chapter.

NOT ENOUGH STRESS?

As mentioned earlier, stress isn't always a bad thing. When Tina Fiandaca attended one of my MHFA training sessions, she had taken the brave and brilliant step of leaving the senior role and business she had worked in for a long time to take a sabbatical. Although she loved the break, what she noticed was that there was very little stress flowing into her dispenser. It gave her a moment of realization that it was time to get back into a new working world, which included a change of career for her. Maybe sometimes there's not enough stress in our lives?

WHEN LIFE GIVES YOU LEMONS ...

Out of difficult and stressful times, good things can come. I took the bitterness of burnout and that stigmatizing comment and discovered a new mission and passion. I learned ways to check in with and support my own mental health. I learned to say yes and no in more helpful ways than ever before.

What can you learn from a full or empty Stress Dispenser, or even one that has overflowed? We keep moving, we take each lesson and experience into the next stage of life. No need to berate yourself if your dispenser gets blocked – make the shift you need and when life gives you lemons, make that delicious lemonade.

THE EXHAUSTION FUNNEL

In May 2020, a couple of months into the pandemic, in the midst of a lockdown, I completed my Mindfulness-Based Cognitive Therapy (MBCT) instructor qualification. It was a tactical self-care move with multiple benefits, not least giving me a non-negotiable reason to turn up for daily mindfulness. It was an international cohort of learners, led by Marion Furr, through The Oxford Mindfulness Centre, within the Department of Psychiatry, University of Oxford, which has been at the forefront of mindfulness research and training since 2008. As such it created an incredibly special and often emotional feeling of global connection as we experienced the world tipping upside down together. I could devote a whole chapter, a whole book in fact, to why MBCT has been a life-changer for me, but instead I'll direct you to the book *Mindfulness: A Practical Guide to Finding Peace in a Frantic World* by Professor Mark Williams and Dr Danny Penman. What I will share are one or two aspects of MBCT, which feel useful to our wider conversation about wellbeing.

In their book, Mark and Danny share the idea of The Exhaustion Funnel to describe how we are pulled into the dark pit of potential burnout when we fail to care for our own psychological and emotional needs. The concept was developed by Professor Marie Asberg, an expert on burnout, at the Karolinska Institute in Stockholm. The World Health Organization recognizes burnout as a modern-day phenomenon, primarily described as chronic workplace stress that has not been successfully managed.

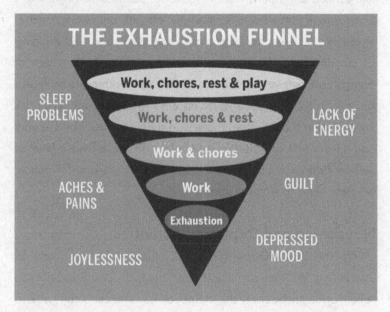

The Exhaustion Funnel

The top circle represents our lives when we lead a balanced and healthy life. As things get busier, many of us tend to give things up to focus on what seems "important" – think back to The Stress Dispenser and our tendency to stop using our helpful coping strategies when stress builds and, worse, turn to unhelpful ones.

The circle narrows, illustrating the narrowing of our lives. Notice the example symptoms and feelings that emerge around the funnel – those shown here are examples (there may be others) and are in no particular order.

When we don't deal with stress, or manage it well, we give up even more of the activities and behaviours that are useful and supportive of our wellbeing and mental health, such as play and rest. The things we give up more easily and quickly are most likely those that nourish us the most but seem to be "optional". The result is that we are increasingly left with only work or other stressors that are often and most likely depleting and draining of our energy and resources, leading to poor sleep, a lack of energy and joylessness, and we are left with nothing to replenish or nourish us. Burnout and illness are the most likely result. It's worth noting that it's often those who might be described as very committed and conscientious people, and those whose level of self-confidence is closely dependent on their work performance, who are likely to suffer burnout.

Nourishing and Depleting Activities

Using The Stress Dispenser and Exhaustion Funnel won't fix everything, but they can act as reminders, check-ins and time to reflect upon and identify the things you can and can't control, and those you can and can't change. At the very least, they can help you bring attention to what you are doing, how you are feeling and coping, and give you the opportunity to explore whether what you are doing is nourishing or depleting your energy. There will always be tasks that we dislike, but that have to be done – at best take a moment to transform and reframe them, or do them more mindfully and put them in the "Mastery" bucket (see below). For example, making a delicious dinner is a necessary act of self-care that you can transform into a "Pleasure" outcome (see below). At worst, simply accept them and choose to do them with a less resentful mood. This book is not about creating the perfect dream life; it's about getting the best out of real life.

TRY THIS ...

Stop. Go on, find five minutes, surely there's five minutes. Write down some of the activities, tasks, responsibilities, fun, purposeful, and well, just general "stuff" you do in an average week or month. Think about what your life looks like, what it's made up of and then go back through the list and ask yourself these two questions:

1. Does this activity lift my mood, give me energy, nourish me, feel good or simply increase my sense of wellbeing and being alive? We call this Nourishing.
2. Does this activity dampen my mood, drain me of energy, or decrease my sense of wellbeing and being alive? We call this Draining or Depleting.

As you work through the list, note whether the activity is N (Nourishing) or D (Depleting or Draining). There's a chance you might want to score some things as both, which is fine and often an interesting moment of reflection.

Now review your list of tasks with their various Ns and Ds assigned to them.

Ask yourself:

- What can I do less of?
- What can I do more of?
- What must I accept?
- What can I control?
- What can I change?
- What can I ask for help with? (This could require an awkward conversation, but we're prepped for that now!)
- What can I share or delegate? (More awkward chat, but putting ourselves first may be essential.)

Ask yourself, what is needed? What do I need and how can I create more space for Ns and minimize and manage the Ds?

It's an exercise you can come back to a few times; you don't have to crack it all in one go. And it will continue to change and evolve, like you!

RADIATORS AND DRAINS

The people in your life can also nourish or deplete you and they can be divided into two camps – Radiators and Drains.

Radiators: These are the people who pump out positivity, warmth, love and kindness, optimism, empathy and enthusiasm; they are interested, interesting and often invested in others. They have the generosity and skill to make you feel good about yourself and bring out the best in you.

Drains: These people are often more glass half empty than full, they struggle to see the positive, they might be self-absorbed, they can zap and deplete your energy.

Begin to notice the amount of time you spend with the Drains versus Radiators in your life. Beware, though, of being overly judgemental; this is simply about your energy management. There's no need to reduce compassion and kindness to others; it is important, though, to apply it to yourself. Be the role model and inspiration to others.

I've heard Oprah reference this exercise, so you know, it's a "thing". My build on it is that I believe we can move from camp to camp, depending on what is happening in our lives, beyond our natural disposition, and so I encourage you to consider *why* someone might be a Drain if you have identified them as such. Are they okay? Do you need to ask them if they need support? Do they need a helping hand to become more of a Radiator? Do remember, though, that in order to keep supporting others, you must find ways to replenish and nourish *your* energy levels. It's about awareness, balance and making shifts when we notice and feel the impact of activities on our energy, wellbeing and overall mental health.

PLEASURE AND MASTERY

There are two types of activities that have been shown to be particularly effective ways to lift the mood: Pleasure and Mastery.

Pleasure Activities
These are the joyful activities that make us feel content and happy, such as phoning a friend for a chat, having a bath, going

for a walk, listening to a podcast, reading, or guilt-free watching a box set or film, and a whole host of examples that are coming up in The M-Plan (see Chapter 9). Pleasure activities don't tend to involve "tasks" and are usually quite relaxing. They can be done on your own and also with others.

What gives you pleasure? Do you do enough of it? Where does it sit in your Nourishing and Draining list of activities? What could you do more of? Go on, give yourself permission, we should all have more pleasure in our lives.

Mastery Activities

These activities give us a sense of achievement, satisfaction and perhaps performance. That job, task or chore even, that we do and enjoy ticking off our list (or the task we do *before* we write the list, that we then put *on* the list so that we have something to tick *off* the list – anyone else?). It's that thing that has a beginning, middle and end or that provides a sense of control and completion. Activities that use our skills, experience and talents – they're things like filling up your food cupboards, getting on top of household admin, clearing and cleaning. They can also be slightly more "downtime" pastimes like playing a musical instrument, dancing for performance, building something, educating yourself or learning something new and, yes, they can be enjoyable and pleasurable, but might be described as less relaxing than pleasure activities.

Mastery can be great for our sense of wellbeing and mood, giving our self-esteem a boost and injecting a sense of accomplishment and actively being well, which can make the biggest difference. Sometimes, when our mood is low, it might even be an easier self-care activity to identify and do compared to those that we describe as pleasurable, but might not be able to find the energy for at that time. It could be the quickest route to self-care.

I asked the iconic singer and performer Beverley Knight MBE about the things she does to look after her mental health and wellbeing and she gave me a spot on example of the important role Mastery activities have in her self-care: "I'm a self-confessed history nerd. I consume books about the Victorian era constantly. I also enjoy listening to social and political discourse, agreeing, disagreeing, changing my mind and changing it back. It's part of my need to learn, to KNOW things. It's my brain workout."

WHAT IS NEEDED?

So, what have we discovered about self-care?

- When our Stress Dispenser is filling up, we may fall into using unhelpful coping strategies. Looking out for our signature stress indicators can help us make shifts toward more helpful coping strategies and toward asking for help using the BRAVE framework.
- An excess of Depleting activities and not so many Nourishing ones, and we're heading to burnout, exhaustion and poor mental health.
- Too many Drains and not enough Radiators in our lives, and we soon have little left to give.
- With no Pleasure activities, we lack a sense of enjoyment, relaxation and perhaps the replenishment of energy.
- With no Mastery activities, our self-esteem, motivation and passion can take a hit.

There's no one magic solution for any of these wellbeing and being well challenges, but becoming aware of them makes a big difference. Almost daily I ask myself "What is needed?" It's simple, it's easy to remember and it helps me to notice what's missing. And once you've got the hang of doing this for yourself, you can pay it forward and use it to support others who may be neglecting their own self-care and be stuck in that bottom right-hand quadrant.

LEADERSHIP IS WITHIN US ALL

In 2019 Gary Booker, Chief Marketing Officer of Rentokil Initial, invited Jonny Benjamin and I to speak at his quarterly team meeting of 50+ people. Gary had dedicated the entire day to the subject of wellbeing. Whilst I know mine and Jonny's stories were impactful, it was Gary who made the greatest difference to the people in the room that day. He shared his own personal experience of a time when a combination of work and personal pressures became overwhelming for him and he realized he needed to address them and ask for support. It was powerful role modelling and a stigma-slaying story for his team to hear; and it was the thing that many of the team talked to me about over drinks at the end of the day.

Mental health really is a leadership issue and it's the personal stories shared that can make the greatest difference. And know this: leadership is within us all.

THE CORNERSTONES OF AWKWARD CONVERSATIONS

Confidence

Self-care keeps your confidence topped up and, better still, growing. When you look after yourself, you are better placed to replenish your energy. In fact, self-care is essential for you to effectively care for others.

Capability

You have a whole heap of new tools to use, not only for your own wellbeing and being well, but also to start a conversation with others you may find yourself supporting. Remember to share, not advise.

Communication

You have more language and definitions – helpful and unhelpful coping strategies, Exhaustion Funnels, Pleasure and Mastery activities and more – to add to your knowledge, support your conversations and strengthen your communication skills.

Compassion

The importance of self-compassion is the message I hope you are courageous enough to take away and put into practice. You can do it.

CHAPTER 9

The M-Plan

*"I think if you can dance and be free and not
embarrassed, you rule the world."*
Amy Poehler

The M-Plan. I made this for ME! Meesh! Michelle Morgan! Mental
Health, Mind Care ... See what I've done there? But it works for
YOU too – you are the ME ... wait, what? Oh, you know what I
mean! But really, please call it whatever you want, just try it.

WHAT AND WHY

I am regularly asked by friends and clients what I do to look after
my mental health and wellbeing, and what I would recommend
to others. It's an interesting question and one that I'd not given
a great deal of thought to (until now). In fact, being asked was
often a bit of an awkward moment; it could propel me back to
feeling a little bit embarrassed or, worse, weak and like I had

failed to look after myself, because I didn't feel like I was doing much for myself that could be described as self-care (I was definitely a bit judgey about the word and idea!).

Over the last few years, though, as I have continued to publicly share my own story, grow Pjoys and continue to deliver mental health training, always pushing myself to find more and better ways to share stories and resources that will make mental health an everyday conversation, I've become increasingly interested in adding to my mission ways to prevent poor mental health from either developing or at least from escalating. And as time has gone on, and I've become more confident, passionate and practised in Owning My Awkward, I've got way more comfortable with the idea of openly talking about how I look after my health – both physical and mental.

GIVING THE MOST AND LIVING THE MOST

I have reached a point where I'm not afraid of self-care. I can say it out loud, not whisper it, without cringing and, hold on to your hats, I'm pretty much at the point of embracing the idea of self-love. Could self-care and self-love be the secret to giving the most, whilst living the most?

Looking after my mental health takes time, attention, discipline and planning, and crucially it's not just about doing one thing; there are a whole host of dos and don'ts that I weave into my day to day, week to week and month to month, even year to year. Oh, yes, and there's also a big slice of forgiveness that I have on standby for each time I fail to do something (or everything) that I know would be good for me and my health.

Here's what I've learned: if I put ME at the centre of my mental health management and self-care, I'm *more likely* to have a healthy life, feel more content and have many more moments of joy. Not only that, I'll be in far better shape to support others and that's really important to me.

TAKING TIME FOR YOURSELF

The good news is that having a holistic approach to looking after ourselves seems to be growing momentum. Kerry Ellis is an English actress and singer, best described as The First Lady of West End Musicals. She shared with me how she has embraced the idea of self-care and reaps the benefits:

Working in the creative industry opens you up to all sorts of uncertain situations; there's lots of anxiety and nerves to deal with and I think we all experience them in some way at some point. The older I get, I have found that having time for myself and taking a moment to give myself some self-care is huge! I use exercise as my therapy; it gives me a moment to just stop and breathe and take stock. It's so important to allow myself this and gives me balance.

YOUR BEINGWELL BUDDY

It's up to you how you use the M-Plan. Adopt and adapt it for YOU – it's a guide, an inspiration and a prompt. Play with it and, please, don't overthink it. Sometimes starting is the hardest part – and the M-Plan gives you six flexible starting points and check-ins to assess and take care of your health and wellbeing:

MOVE | MEDITATE | MAKE | MEET
MEANING | MINDSET

Think of the M-Plan as your Beingwell Buddy. Wellbeing is your state. Being Well is all about action.

Used alongside the M-Plan are some additional principles that I've called the The Six Supports, which I know I need to have covered to protect my mental health, confidence and wellbeing.

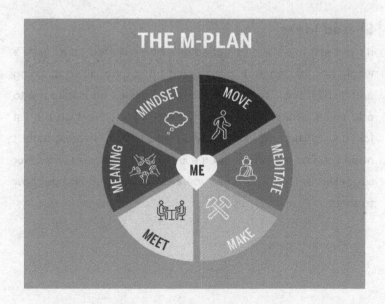

The Ms are flexible and freeing, in that they can be interpreted in a variety of ways to work for you. You might find some more appealing; some might already be a natural part of your day, week, month. Some might cross over – e.g. one person's MOVE might be running, whereas another's running is a form of MEDITATION. Interpret them however you like – if it works for you, it works!

Use the Ms alongside the tools from Chapter 8 – The Stress Dispenser, Exhaustion Funnel, the Nourishing and Depleting, and Pleasure and Mastery exercises. The combination of these will help you answer my favourite question, and I hope, soon to be yours – "What is needed?" What do you need right now? What do you need more of? Less of? What could you try? What would happen if you tried? Try using the Four Steps To Owning Your Awkward (see page 80) to help get you in the right frame of mind.

Shared Ideas

It's not just my Ms in this chapter – I've included ideas from a whole host of generous people and I find them all so touching and inspirational. They really make me smile and inspire me to add some different ideas to my own M-Plan. Next on the list for me are dancing like a jellyfish and having a forest bath! I hope you find the same – let me know your favourites and other suggestions. Go to www.ownyourawkward.com to find out how to share.

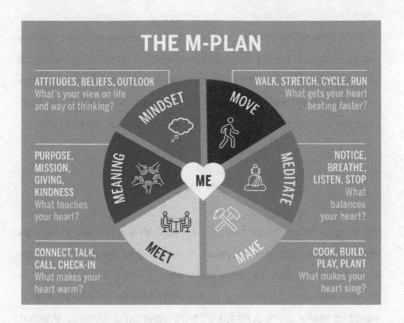

A Note About Music

A couple of people pointed out that I had missed MUSIC. Fair comment. Except I didn't. The Ms are flexible and, for me, music can be a response to a few of the Ms ... and I wanted to see if it was the same for others (it seems to be, as you'll see). Whether dancing to music (MOVE), listening to music (MEDITATE), making music (MAKE), listening and watching music together (MEET), the gift of music to others (MEANING) or listening to a favourite motivational track (MINDSET) – I'll have Youngblood Brass Band, *Brooklyn* (infectious and the BEST) to kick things off, thanks... it works for each of the Ms in its own wonderful way. Music should run through our lives, and it certainly runs through mine.

Nihal Arthanayake describes the role of music to support his mental health so eloquently (after pointing out that I missed out music out of the Ms, so this one's going out to you Nihal):

You have missed out music, which is a massive part of allowing me to escape from my thoughts and revel in something beautiful and emotional. I find that listening to new songs that enlighten and inspire me make me feel lighter and more alive. To lose yourself in a song is psychological, spiritual and physical.

MOVE

What gets your heart beating faster? We need to move, as best we can, for our physical, mental and emotional health and wellbeing, but it's not always easy. I find the word exercise pressurized and off-putting ... a quick reframe to MOVE and it starts to make more sense, be more open and inviting. We can move in so many different ways, can't we? Exercise sounds like a chore, whereas MOVE sounds more joyful. For me, it's simply about walking, ideally with my dog (furry son), Teddy.

I am a fan of working out, whether the gym is open or not. Rain or shine, I'll be lifting, getting my heart rate up and sweating. Feels great. I have weights and resistance bands at home. After the workout I get into a bath of freezing water to help inflammation, circulation, as well as sharpening my focus. Trust me. You know you're alive after that!
Beverley Knight MBE
Musical Artist

After almost two years of seeing the world in black and white, due to Postnatal Depression, I started running again to see if I could improve my physical health. Run by gradual run, the colour started to fade back in. As each week went by, I found myself more and more surprised at just how bad I had felt the week before, and more able to feel excitement about the future. For me, it's the most important tool in my mental health locker. I know I need to do it in the morning as that's the best time for me to process and plan my working day. I know I need to listen to music that makes me happy. I know I need to hear my heart beating loudly. I can't say that I see in technicolour all the time now, but when I feel the colour start to fade, I Move, Move, Move.

Alexandra Goat

CEO Livity

MOVE is meditation for me on many levels. Swimming for example – the steady motion, the rhythm, the breathing, the quietening of the mind. I completed a free-diving course recently and in the early stages of learning about static apnea I was so surprised to find out how much breathing had an effect on me even though I had been practising "belly breathing" for a few years.

Stormie Mills

Artist

Regular movement keeps me sane and a morning walk or practising yoga, especially in nature, brings me home to a healthy place of "What's here when I'm not looking for what's not here?" At the same time, I think rest is sorely underrated

in our culture and if it's helpful, then rest can be just as heal-ing, if not more so, than movement.
Lelly Aldworth
Yoga Teacher

What does it mean to move? For me it's the idea that movement starts from the inside out. A breath, a feeling, that follows and shifts the body in space and time. Our bod-ies carry their own natural rhythms. Think about the beat of your heart or the pulse of blood racing through your veins. In stillness you can feel the pace that your body naturally wants to take on. There is an exercise that I allow my body to move through each day, which is starting still and allowing my in-hale to move my body in one way then the exhale to move in the next way. I like to have the movements feel never-ending and infinite. There is no way to really describe what this is going to look like as each day it will take a different form, but if you would like to try it, maybe think about a jellyfish pulsating through water and let that image move from your mind into your breath and then your body.
Aicha McKenzie
Breath Coach and Founder of AMCK

My go-to move come rain or shine is cycling in my local park. I go there to do my best thinking. I get to listen to new albums on little bike speakers.
Bejay Mulenga
Founder of Supa Network

Dance! Dance! Dance!
Jenny Tillotson
Founder, eScent

I am SUCH a big champion of walking. I think when talking about mental health (and what I call brain care), it can become so easy to overcomplicate things, but the way I use movement is to stack so many great behaviours on top of one another and go from there. For example, I start my day with a daily walk (around 60–90 minutes) and depending on what day it is, and what I have to do, I'll listen to a podcast or audiobook, have a phone call/walking meeting, soak in the atmosphere and nature around me. I always try to spend at least ten minutes of it just silently observing my surroundings mindfully – and I do it rain or shine. Movement and health isn't all about that 60-minute HIIT session, just ten minutes of walking a day is enough to transform it!
Dan Murray-Serter
Co-founder, Heights

20 MOVES

Cycling. Football. Hula–Hooping. Skipping.
Yoga. Basketball. Netball.
Dancing (whether like a jellyfish or not). Stretching.
Weightlifting. Walking. Pilates. Hockey. Circuit
training. Climbing. Swimming. Rambling. Skating.
Playing with your dog. Tai Chi.

MEDITATE

What calms your heart? How can you stop, breathe, notice, connect, find calm? How can you bring some peace and stillness to your chittering-chattering mind and even a sense of regained control or acceptance? How can you create space to cultivate your intuition? How can you be mindful, aware and present? Meditation and mindfulness are recovery for the mind. Often people think and say that they can't meditate. The first step is to be kind to yourself; it's not about being able to do it or being good at it; it's about creating a space that gives you, and perhaps your body and mind, a gentle break or a chance to reconnect with yourself. No need to overthink it! When your mind wanders, and 100% guaranteed it will, all you need to do is notice and acknowledge this and gently walk your attention back to your breath or the activity you are doing. And keep doing it, over and over. I regularly follow the principles of Mindfulness-Based Cognitive Therapy (MBCT). Keep in mind, too, that meditation doesn't have to mean sitting in a formal pose – there are many informal ways to be meditative.

> *I heard the ADHD brain described as a Ferrari brain with bicycle brakes. That pretty much describes me. Yoga, meditation and breathing are essential to me for slowing myself down. When I find it hard, which I do all the time, I know it's because I need it. It's incredibly powerful to have that self-awareness – I wish I'd had it 20 years ago!*
> **Jo Davey**
> Talent Director

I am a CALM App user and I've done Headspace too. I have found the focus on breathing so useful throughout my life. I love mindful moments and find nature powerful for that. We live near woods and to stop and touch bark, listen to the sounds, watch a bird – I mean stop and really watch it – will snap you into the moment. I am a 100% believer in the power of the Japanese idea of Shinrin-Yoku – 'Forest bathing', which means taking in the forest atmosphere as you walk.

Jez Felwick

Founder, The Bowler Food Truck and Swaadish Curry Sauces

Meditation can look like a lot of things for me. When my daughter was born and I didn't have time to sit down to meditate, I had a "foot awareness practice". I would just feel into my feet at any given moment and feel more present, more grounded and more alive. I get so much out of sitting down to meditate – 40 minutes seems to be the magic amount for me. I think Jon Kabat-Zinn, the mindfulness expert, recommends that amount of time for meditation to have a potent effect and that has been true for me.

Chrissie Nicholson

Director of Sustainability and Purpose, Pjoys

Meditation has been hugely beneficial to my mental health. It's taken a while for me to fully understand and embrace it, first coming to it in my mid-20s but struggling to grasp it properly. Years of reading and learning about it have helped me to apply it to my life. Now I really notice the benefits of meditating, and the impact it has on my wellbeing when I stop practising. The key to meditation, for me, is self-compassion. Once you're able to unlock this, a whole new world can open up for you.

Jonny Benjamin MBE

Founder, Beyond, author and mental health campaigner

Over the last year I have moved from straight meditation sat on the seat to Bath Meditation during a bath soak with salts – I've been enjoying the relaxation and energy from the heat of the bath.

Bejay Mulenga

Founder, Supa Network

I have learned from my husband, James, that taking time to meditate every day is important. Every morning I go into my garden, stand on the grass in bare feet and breathe and stretch. It's known as grounding, or earthing. It's plugging into the ecology of which we are all a part.

Beverley Knight MBE

Musical Artist

I started to learn to meditate when I came off meds in 2019. I used the Waking Up App, which taught me how to breathe (and to stop holding my breath). This is a first step – I'm still a beginner!"

Jenny Tillotson MBE

Founder, eScent

Finding the balance between meditation and movement is summed up beautifully in The Idiot's Complete Guide to Yoga where it says "Feeling great? Meditate. Feeling down? Move around".

Lelly Aldworth

Yoga Teacher

20 MEDITATES

Mindfulness sitting practice. Playing a musical instrument.
Listening to a podcast (or simply noises)
with your full attention.
Walking and noticing on purpose. Mindful movement.
Listening to music. Reading.
Having a sound bath. Guided meditation.
Qigong meditation. Body scan. Yoga Nidra.
Listening to the birds and other wildlife. Tai Chi.
Mindful washing-up.
Mantra meditation. @lost_and_left_ project.
Zen meditation. Cutting vegetables and cooking mindfully.
Colouring.

MAKE

What makes your heart sing? We have an innate need as human beings to "make", to use our hands, our bodies and, yet, in the modern world many of us just don't seem to have the time or inclination and energy to make things. The making that we *have* to do can feel like a chore, not something joyful or nourishing. During the Covid-19 pandemic we had more time and there was a lot more making all around as people taught themselves new skills or picked up arts and crafts once more or for the first time (and many didn't and that's okay too!). In the UK there was a mass-making of sourdough bread and then banana bread; it was something we could do for ourselves and others, something quite mindful perhaps to calm a chattering head (MEDITATE!), skilful and with a sense of mastery (ah, MASTERY there it is!), with a successful and tasty outcome (PLEASURE) – and for those baking fails, it was an opportunity to learn and have another go. My MAKE is gardening; making our outside space colourful, calm and alive gives me a great sense of pleasure and also a bit of mastery when I tackle the weeds and learn about how to keep flowers and plants alive (or even get them to grow in the first place).

@_LOST_AND_LEFT

Remi and I started a part MEDITATE, part MAKE mindfulness project – @Lost_and_Left_ on Instagram – during London's first lockdown, in early 2020, as part of our daily "move". I like to describe it as a noticing project, as it only works if you have your eyes open and are fully aware. It started years ago;

I couldn't see a lone shoe, on a pavement, in the road, on the side of the motorway, without wondering: Who? Why? When? Where's the other one? For decades I'd wonder, just to myself. Then I began to say it out loud to Remi. Well, during the pandemic was the moment I decided to start capturing pictures of random shoes I noticed. Remi joined in and then we began seeing other items, some looked as though they had been lost, some increasingly were left, as people used the extra time at home to tidy, sort, clear and chuck out. It's fun and funny, it's creative, it's playful and it helps us receive the benefits of being present as we're out and about with, as my BFF Lulu encourages, "our heads up and eyes looking out" rather than stuck in our phones or caught up in our thoughts.

Making good food for yourself or others has a special warmth and love to it, along with a sense of agency when anything else seems like all too much.
Lelly Aldworth
Yoga Teacher

There are certain making activities where I can enter a flow state. Time warps, you can be totally fixated on the make in hand. The self-talk ceases and you have clarity, I love it. Making music and playing the guitar badly is one for me, as is playing records, music and mixing. Cooking is another, as is gardening.
Jez Felwick
Founder, The Bowler Food Truck & Swaadish Curry Sauces

Everyone can make and create; it is about the process as much as the outcome. The important thing is to make for your sake and not for likes on social media. I love everything crafty and spent my childhood learning how to knit one week, and then make candles the next, but my biggest creative output happens in the kitchen. From a young age I found that being in the kitchen made me so content. I liked the meditative action of kneading or washing up, but I also liked having a final outcome that could feed me, and feed others. Essentially being in the kitchen allows me to go into my own little world where I can switch off from all the stresses of life.

David Atherton

Food writer, health adviser, charity worker and *The Great British Bake Off* winner

My experience of mental ill-health has inspired me to do something radically positive with my life and for my kids. For people like myself with poor mental health, I have made and patented a solution called eScent, to help with the crippling impact of anxiety and to help people breathe better. An intelligent system detects an increase in stress and then a personalized scent is delivered as a diffused sensory "Bubble" and intervention for mental distress, all through the ancient art of perfumery married with emerging technologies and wearable AI-powered scent technology platform.

Jenny Tillotson

Founder, eScent

I am a comedian. I am a performer. During the first part of lockdown my mental health suffered. Then I started doing online shows. My wife Amelia and I created an online game show, which we did on Zoom. It gave me focus; I was creating and using my skill set and achieving the satisfaction of putting on a good show. That show and the other online stand-up shows I did pulled me out of a dark funk. Dark Funk being the worst of the Daft Punk tribute bands.

Jarred Christmas

Comedian

For me it's definitely MAKE! I make my art, I make food, I make music and I do my best to make my family happy and safe and all of that making supports my wellbeing.

Remi Rough

Artist

20 MAKES

Make music. Make tunes. Make nutritious and delicious meals. Arrange window boxes with flowers and plants. Grow vegetables. Build a sandcastle. Play with Lego. Do a modelling kit. Do a jigsaw. Paint or colour. Write a story. Practical or creative home improvements (pleasurable ones). Make a film. Write a song. Gardening. Make a vision board. Make your living space tidy and ordered. Make a mess. Make or mend your clothes. Build a fire and toast marshmallows.

MEET

What connections warm your heart? As with MAKE, and as we found out earlier in this book, we have a natural need for belonging and above all else, perhaps, love. Sometimes it's the smallest of actions that can make the greatest difference. When we are with others we have a greater sense of connection and communication, conversation and engagement, kindness and, of course, compassion. Giving someone our attention offers connection and, as we've learned, can be achieved even in the silence. Whilst being more of an introvert than extrovert, I love being with people. I've learned, though, that I need to be super mindful of whom, where and how often, watching out for too much time with the Drains, seeking out the Radiators and giving myself recovery time to be quiet and ensure I don't overcommit, which is a discipline of its own.

> I go to comedy nights twice a month minimum, I meet my cousins or siblings to watch comedies and documentaries. I love lighthearted stories that make me laugh.
> **Bejay Mulenga**
> Founder Supa Network

> Friends and family ... human contact, it's what the time on this planet is surely all about and sharing experiences good, bad and ugly. My friends care, listen and help, so will yours, even if you don't think they will. I sometimes think that I don't want to burden my mates with heavy

thoughts or worries, but just converting the thoughts into words can shift the mindset. I am lucky and have great mates who ask about feelings and I now try to ask people how they are really feeling, to give a chance and space to share and listen.

Jez Felwick

Founder, The Bowler Food Truck and Swaadish Curry Sauces

My Mermaids swimming group, joining the gym, walking Ziggy ... all in a new place when I moved to the sea. Just being brave enough to get out there, on my own and meet new people.

Meg Mathews

Founder, Meg's Menopause

I do my best thinking and self-analysis out loud by meeting and connecting with those I love and respect. When I feel things getting out of control, I need to get it off my chest as often I answer my own questions and diminish my own fears by speaking them out loud. I tend to rotate who I speak to at different emotional times.

Jess Butcher

Entrepreneur and Business Adviser

Meeting my younger self who really struggled and suffered and not only meeting him, but loving him, caring for him, being compassionate to him and making him feel like he is connected to me. It was my younger self creating an alarm in my system and that's who I had to meet to really heal from my mental health challenges and reassure him, using my adult self, the competent doctor in me.

Dr Russ

Doctor, comedian and author

Never underestimate the power of a hug.

Tyrone Joseph

Product Development Manager, Tate

20 MEETS

Send a card or a letter. Send a short text to say hi.
Make a phone call. Arrange some flowers through the post or deliver them unannounced. Have a chat in a queue.
Make some small talk with the person serving you in the shop or restaurant. Don't be afraid of deep talk. Join a community group. Learn something new that involves other people.
Join a choir. Join a walking group or a charity challenge.
Explore potential hobbies. Suggest a "walkie talkie" with a co-worker. Knock on your neighbour's door.
Do some volunteering. Be the one to get your friends together. Go on a date night. Go to that work event you're not sure about. Join a sports group. Tell someone you love them, tell them why you love them.

MEANING

What touches your heart? We all need a sense of meaning in our lives. What is your mission or purpose? It doesn't matter how big or small and it doesn't have to be fixed. MEANING can be found through our work, at home, in our community. It can be an idea or doing something differently that has an impact. Meaning can be generated and inspired; it can be found in the tiniest of actions and experiences. It can be as simple as checking in on a neighbour, supporting a good cause through your work, putting greater purpose and social impact at the heart of your business, getting more involved in your child's school life. Open yourself to the idea of having meaning and it will come. I receive most of my meaning through the work I do, the businesses I create and lead and the organizations I support and cheerlead, like being an Ambassador for MHFA England.

Meaning is purpose to me. I don't need to find the meaning of life, but its purpose for me while I am still alive. This often comes to me by the result of my personal interactions and the sense I get from serving others, I am often seeking something bigger than my capacity to make me feel useful and alive.
Carlos Mare
Sculptor, Curator, Scholar

I have been involved in a few charitable activities and find that helping others in any small way gives meaning and purpose beyond working for cash. It definitely boosts your

self-esteem knowing that you've done something and made a difference, however small.
Jez Felwick
Founder, The Bowler Food Truck and Swaadish Curry Sauces

I have spent the last couple of years building a life I don't want to escape from, so naturally for me, everything has meaning. I decided I wanted to live every day like I am on holiday. It sounds simple but it means my career, my friendships, my hobbies, what I watch, listen to and read all have intention. I choose to be mentally, soulfully and physically well every day; in making that choice it dictates my actions.
Natalie Campbell
CEO, Belu Water

To nurture a sense of meaning in my life is putting my family first, feeling grateful, socializing with friends.
Lindsay King
Teacher

Having a meaningful conversation and exchange with someone who really gets you is such a nourishing balm for the soul.
Lelly Aldworth
Yoga Teacher

For me, it's important to be inspired by my work, and I am lucky to work in an industry that I love. There are often stressful days and moments when I feel overwhelmed or lose my confidence, but our shared mission at the gallery to help people find themselves in art keeps me grounded."

Jen Scott

Director, Dulwich Picture Gallery, London

Music is everything to me. The ultimate joy giver. I was taught by my parents to believe that my higher purpose is to be an agent for change and progression, using the music gifts I was handed at birth. To that end I try to use it through the charities I support to meet that higher purpose. That gives my existence meaning to me.

Beverley Knight MBE

Musical Artist

20 MEANINGS

Work, charity, gifting, giving, listening,
connecting, channelling a gift to give others' pleasure,
kindness, gratitude, caring, talking, volunteering,
vocational, spiritual, creating a business, a charity,
a community group, lobbying, educating,
making a difference big or small.

MINDSET

How we view and think about situations, opportunities and challenges, the world even, depends a great deal on our MINDSET, beliefs and approach to life. Whilst much of our mindset is shaped by our old friend the Frame of Reference (see page 48), we can nurture our mindset, we can choose to explore and evolve it. For example, we might adopt techniques to move from a fixed mindset – "I can't change who I am" to a growth mindset – "I'm a work in progress and have the ability to evolve and change". It's kind of how our Transformative questions work in the Four Steps To Owning Your Awkward (see page 80). Having a positive or, better still, growth mindset can contribute enormously to the quality and state of our mental health.

SELF-TALK

Sara Milne Rowe, author of *The SHED Method*, coached me and the team in the very early days of Livity and one of her many gifts is helping people make choices that help them to be who they want and achieve what they want. She explained:

Mindset, for me, is about how you are talking to yourself, what you are saying, when you are saying it and in what tone. Asking yourself, would I say that to my best friend?

Mindset can have a heaviness about it, so how about we take a playful approach to nurturing it ... ask yourself,

> *what's my experiment today, to find out more about me? What's going to be encouraging for me, what will up my motivation, meaning and purpose, but that's not a deal-breaker? This is what I call "Energy Self-Talk", it's mindful and deliberate. I have post-it notes all over my walls with the things I want to say to myself. The place you get confidence from is the past. Confidence is an output not a state, so when those good, positive and proud moments happen, recognize them, bank them, put them in your Yay Book or Trophy Cabinet and come back to them often. Place attention and energy on what is working for you, however small and whoever you are."*

I love the idea of "The Yay Book", because whilst writing is such a therapeutic outlet for me, I sometimes feel journalling is tinged with a slightly more sombre vibe. I love the idea of noting those proud, yay moments.

I support a positive mindset by being honest and using comparisons. If today is a "bad day", then I express how fortunate I know I am to have many days that are great days, and that tomorrow might be better.
Dan Murray-Serter
Co-founder, Heights

To look after myself I go beyond a positivity mindset and instead focus on being calm and grounded in the reality of the moment. Most stress is tied to what happened (the past) and what ifs (future); I don't let the thoughts escalate by bringing joy, bliss or simply contentment into the current moment I am experiencing.

Natalie Campbell

CEO, Belu Water

I am luckily, pretty positive as a default and have found that the entrepreneurial types tend to be. I have had some tragic events happen in recent years and found being aware of the fragility of life can really help shape a positive, grab-life mindset. You really might be dead tomorrow, or in a minute. Your time is the most valuable thing you have, trade it wisely.

Jez Felwick

Founder, The Bowler Food Truck & Swaadish Curry Sauces

Mindset is what I focus on most actively whenever I start to feel overwhelmed or feel the "demons" rushing in shouting "not good enough", "not this enough, not that enough". I have to actively put myself in a position of greater perspective, forcing myself to step out of myself and get things back into focus, asking myself "In the broader scale of things, does this matter? Will it matter? What's the worse that could happen?" The answers are typically "No", "No" and "Not the end of the world".

Jess Butcher

Entrepreneur and Business Adviser

I've learned to remind myself that "thoughts are not facts". I try to remind myself of this when I feel my anxiety is triggered as it's often thoughts and even paranoia that take over first.

Susie Shaw

Founder, Mind Over Cancer, counsellor and MHFA instructor

Reset, reset, reset every day. I have learned that mindset is not a fixed state that even at my lowest I can reset.

Carlos Mare

Sculptor, Curator, Scholar

I have a couple of mantras. When out walking I tell myself "look up and out" and when my day feels a challenge "be the best you can be today".

Lindsay King

Teacher

20 MINDSETS

Ask yourself Transformative questions (see page 82) – Reframe. Set goals, short-term or long-term. Make a visualization board of how you want your life to look. Create moments of reflection to check in with your mindset and mood. Choose your mood. Get a coach. Ask a friend to be your accountability buddy (work, life or self-care). Try talking therapies. Explore Cognitive Behavioural

Therapy. Have a go at Mindfulness-Based Cognitive Therapy (with me!). Notice your inner narrative and try switching to positive self-talk. Assess what is depleting your energy and mindset. Do the Nourishing exercise (see page 183). Consider the Drains and Radiators in your life (see page 184). Check how you are talking to yourself. Set a positive mantra. Start a Yay book. Ask yourself what is needed. Give yourself permission to do what you need to do. Be kind to yourself.

NO PRESSURE!

There's an important point to be made, especially if you are perhaps feeling a sense of overwhelm and asking yourself (or me), "How on earth can I fit all these things into my day to day, week to week even?" There's a lot here. In fact, the point was made beautifully by Jez when he shared his Ms with me, "All of the Ms resonate completely with me. One thing I want to say though is that I fail regularly to keep on top of actioning some of these, BUT I have realized, now, that this is okay! For example, I'm useless at meditation, but I still know it's beneficial even when I can't master it."

Three is the Magic Number

To build on Jez's point, there's no way I can tick each M on a daily or even weekly basis. Some don't get a look in for more than a month. At other times I can feel the benefits of trying my best to incorporate them into my life, sometimes naturally if I'm super lucky. We can be so hard on ourselves and, let's face it, no day or week is the same. It's the act of being kind to ourselves, when either we make time (well done, pat on the back for super self-care) or when we forget, we get distracted, can't be bothered or really don't have time. Remember, though, just because you didn't do it today or this week, doesn't mean you can't do it tomorrow or next week. That's the discipline – forgiving yourself and trying tomorrow, like Carlos Mare says, "reset, reset, reset". Maybe set yourself a target of three Ms per day, or week, if that is your best right now. As Lindsay shared, "When my day feels a challenge my mantra is 'be the best you can be today'."

THE SIX SUPPORTS

There are some additional strands of support that help me manage my mental health. No, they don't begin with M, but lucky for me and the way my brain is wired, they do begin with S – Stupendous! Look, I need every trick possible to look after my mental health. I'd describe The Six Supports as the scaffolding to The M-Plan, my wellbeing and my being well. They are:

SLEEP | SUSTENANCE | SECURITY | SEX STRUCTURE | SPONTANEITY

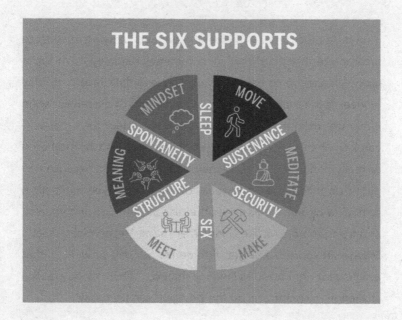

Sleep

The importance of sleep is underestimated, although the good news is that there's more and more evidence emerging that promotes the benefits of having the right amount (for you) of quality sleep, both for your physical and mental health. Essentially quality sleep helps make your brain rest and work properly. Here are some tips that might help:

- Find the bedtime and wake-up times that best suit you.
- Turn screens and blue lights on devices off at least an hour before bedtime.
- Try not to eat too much too close to bedtime.
- Learn how caffeine can impact your sleep.
- Create winding-down rituals and signals.
- Have a consistency to your sleep times and habits.

Sustenance

Food, water, nourishment, energy – the key elements that sustain our lives. What we put (or don't put) in our bodies can affect and impact our health, physically, mentally and emotionally. Like with sleep, there is increasing evidence of the importance of the relationship between our gut and brain health and so it is worth thinking about and paying attention to the food, drinks, vitamins and supplements we choose to sustain us. There are different approaches – find the school of thought that is best for you. Follow @catherine_arnold_ nutrition on Instagram for inspiration.

Security

For me this manifests itself in terms of financial security, swiftly extending to the security of my family beyond finances. Security is also about being free from feelings of anxiety and so all of those Ms play an important role. Mindset, the tools and techniques that I've learned through having therapy, and LOADS of self-development and self-care are important for helping me gain perspective in the moments I fall into overthinking and catastrophizing. Security is about feeling like I'm living in a safe space to be myself, in safe relationships, doing work that feels right for me, with sight of income flowing in – interestingly it doesn't dampen my entrepreneurial spirit and need to not be shackled to a job working for someone else. Maybe it should. Maybe it will one day! After all, I'm a work in progress.

Sex

If I'm honest, I'm Owning My Awkward right now to include the importance of sex. I'm blushing. But if I can't feel awkward here, where can I? To feel attractive, wanted, desired, touched, held, loved and have fun that creates connection in an intimate way is an important part of life, mental health and wellbeing. It's an aspect of life that is vulnerable in so many ways. If your self-esteem and confidence are low, it can affect how you feel about yourself, someone else and your libido in general. On the plus side, it can comfort you, help get you out of your head, or into a different place in your head and bring a great big smile to your face (or whatever your sex face is – gulp, more awkward). Talking about it can be awkward, but like mental health conversations, the benefits outweigh the awkward. And of course there's Masturbation, another M!

Structure

I have resisted structure for so much of my life, but I do know that having *some* in my day to day, week to week, is helpful, no critical, to looking after myself, especially my mental health and sense of wellbeing. Structure means I do the M-Plan, that I check in with The Six Supports. It means I take my medication, my supplements, make nourishing food and prioritize the important things in my life. Structure helps me be organized and feel on top of things and it helps me to say "No" when I need to and saying "No" helps me to do more of the things that I want to do.

Spontaneity

What can I say? I know this sounds like a contradiction, but I'm complicated! Yes, structure is an important aspect of looking after my overall health and wellbeing. As long as I start with structure and keep coming back to it, I can enjoy moments of spontaneity, rather than getting horribly lost for months down wormholes. I have often described myself as a compliant introverted extrovert, who likes to rebel. I benefit from structure and continuity, then there are the times (quite regularly) when boredom hits me and that's when breaking the status quo can be beneficial to me.

And that's that. The Ms and the Ss that work to keep me and my physical, mental and emotional health in check. Prompts, reminders, inspiration, I embrace them all with both a sense of structure and spontaneity. With a die-hard commitment and equal amounts of forgiveness when I fail to embrace them, or they're just not seemingly that useful. Because we now know that life isn't black and white, we know that it's up and down, we're clear that our mental health isn't fixed, we all have it, it moves. And try yes, try your best, but go easy on yourself too.

THE CORNERSTONES OF AWKWARD CONVERSATIONS

Confidence

Engage with The M-Plan and The Six Supports and you'll soon have more conversation starters and solutions in your toolkit to share, as well as a whole host of ideas and actions for taking better care of your own mental health. All of this will add to your overall confidence for talking about mental health and being well.

Capability

Whilst some might say practice makes perfect, you really don't have to be super talented or great at any of these inspirations and activities. Approach The M-Plan playfully. Be curious, give it a go. It's good for our mental health to try to learn different things.

Communication

The M-Plan and The Six Supports will give you loads to talk about. Share what works to support your overall mental health and find out what works for others.

Compassion

Making your own mental health and self-care a priority is not only an act of self-compassion, it tops you up and provides you with more room to be compassionate to others. Do what you can, when you can.

CHAPTER 10

Awkward is Your Greatest Asset

"I want to feel my life whilst I'm in it."

Meryl Streep

There are multiple reasons I wanted to write this book. First and foremost, my mission, at this moment in my life, truly, is to make mental health an easier and everyday conversation. I believe I have a role to play – remember "Survivors Mission" in Chapter 7? This book extends and amplifies my day-to-day work and service to others and I am enormously grateful to have added the medium of writing to my portfolio of training, speaking and pyjama-wearing formats and platforms. To reach more people and share what I've learned about mental health – mountains of information that I wish I'd known long before I actually ever did – really blimmin' excites me. To share the frameworks I've designed and created to help make that information and knowledge more accessible and easier to digest and use, makes my head spin and my heart swell.

Secondly, in a noisy world, this book has given me something that I've often struggled to find, project or value – and that is my voice. And now my voice is proudly here, in its own space, a place that anyone and everyone is invited into, and that I hope will be in tune and melodious for many, whilst knowing also that it won't be for everyone and that's okay. We all need to find our own choir. The same can be said for having awkward conversations. Some conversations, once you've pushed on through the awkward will go swimmingly, pitch perfect; others, well, you'll find yourself sinking, sometimes a little, very occasionally a lot, regretting having even started them as they play out, with the occasional bum note, or more awkwardly, a cacophony of wrong notes. This is life. It's okay. Please don't let the conversations that don't go so well stop you from trying again.

Thirdly, I talk to a lot of people about mental health, a lot of the time, and what I've noticed, is that for me, whilst 100% acknowledging the global conversation-stopping problem that is "stigma", it is rarely difficult to get people talking about mental health and to gather anecdotes, stories, experiences, sadness, hopefulness and more, from all kinds of people, from all walks of life, and that gives me hope and a belief that the ideas in this book are worth sharing and amplifying. I have no special powers, I have simply learned to Own My Awkward and when I own mine, other people seem to own theirs more easily, and talk.

This book was nearly called "It's Not Awkward!" as the (slightly shouty) challenge and response to being told "It's a bit awkward when you talk about your mental health Michelle", as I was burning out and slipping further into a deep hole of unwellness and depression. On the other side of that time and remark, when I did start talking about my mental health once more, I had a sense that it wasn't really so awkward, after all I was talking about it a lot. Coining the title "It's Not Awkward!" had felt like a revelation to me. It felt like *that* was the insight and stigma-smashing message that I needed to take out to the world – that it didn't need to be, and now wasn't for me, awkward talking about my mental health. But I had a niggle that I was going in the wrong direction, and it turns out the niggle was right (always listen to those messengers of intuition!). One morning I woke up and saw a Brené Brown Instagram post that simply said "Stay Awkward!" and that was the actual moment of revelation. Of course, it *is* awkward talking about mental health, it's *still* awkward for me, and let's face it, I talk about it *all* the time and yes, it's almost *always* awkward, but it's how I have learned to manage, value and love my awkwardness, own it even, that makes it something I can do more easily these days. It *is* still awkward though. Saying "It's Not Awkward!" was just me shouting, on my own, still hurt, still angry, still embarrassed and wounded by words that had, at the very least, been used carelessly and thoughtlessly, or at the very worst been used as weapons to make me feel small and controlled.

"Own Your Awkward" is me taking ownership of those weaponized words and recalibrating them into a rallying cry, not just for me, for us all. It's an encouragement, a celebration, and something to be proud of when you do it. It's about belonging, connection, kindness and help. It can even bring smiles, warmth and laughter. Maybe it's a movement, a club, a community or perhaps it's just an idea that a whole lot of us can gather around and give flight to. It's recovery and it is hope. And look, let's face it, when Brené Brown says stay awkward, you stay awkward.

WHAT NEXT?

"How are you? How are you really?" Keep asking that question and you'll keep getting better and more confident at it. Keep on answering the question too. And if you've not yet asked someone how they are doing, or if they need some support, you're pretty much ready to go, to start that conversation and offer someone help, or indeed ask for help if you need it. There's never a perfect moment for your first knowingly awkward conversation and whilst the more you do it, the easier it will become, maybe we need to also accept that it's always going to remain a little bit uncomfortable, because we care, and that's a good kind of awkward.

IT TAKES SUN AND RAIN TO MAKE A RAINBOW

What makes us awkward also makes us brilliant and in tune with others – and the things holding us back can also be the things that propel us forward. Sometimes recovery benefits from minor changes, baby steps, achievable goals and at other times it needs more of a major move, perhaps changing careers, companies and countries even. I organized my recovery around a newly found mission and purpose, creativity and launching a new entrepreneurial venture, Pjoys – PJs with Purpose. My school friend Kate Higham pours her experience and challenges of mental ill-health, not only into making her beautiful jewellery and pottery, but also into supporting others. She told me:

Mental illness has been the making of me. I've had to do the work others fear to tread. I cannot remember much of the dark days, but I know well the challenge of getting through them and, as such, the unseen struggle has bred a rather strong and grounded person, who has along the way tried to listen to, and empower and encourage, other souls who have bravely opened up to me. I hope one day having a "mental health check" is as common as having an "eye health check".

THE CORNERSTONES OF
AWKWARD CONVERSATIONS
A SUMMARY

Confidence

Information, knowledge about mental health, mental ill-health and diagnosis are all confidence boosters and stigma-smashing assets, plus you have the SENSE framework for offering help. Now to practise, to go for it, to just plain do it, start a conversation, and feel the response, along the way noting what went well or what you would do differently next time. If it didn't *feel* like a great conversation, that doesn't mean it wasn't helpful or impactful. Don't be hard on yourself. Congratulate yourself for having the courage to offer help. The great thing about confidence is that it is a lifelong work in progress; you can continue to grow it.

You also understand that true fear is a survival signal that sounds *only* in the presence of danger, and that worry is manufactured and a waste of time. You have the evidence and encouragement to listen to your intuition and know that when you feel a hesitation about doing something, it might be an indicator to do it.

The BRAVE framework gives you the courage to have a conversation with yourself and ask for help, and the strength to look after yourself and your own mental health, to put yourself first, to put your hand up when you are struggling, whenever and wherever. It's the best and bravest thing to do, for you, but also for those around you, who care about you, and they do. You are not a burden, you're a beautiful human being who will experience the ups and downs of life. Remember that recovery is the most likely outcome, and that will come sooner when you talk about how you are feeling and coping and when you ask for support. If you are stuck in the bottom right-hand quadrant of the Mental Health Continuum, please be BRAVE and talk to someone you trust.

Because you've learned about our need to socially belong, we can reframe our hesitation to ask for help knowing that the person we're asking for help from is going to get so much from giving you support. Give Give Get!

Capability

The Frame of Reference, the Mental Health Continuum, the Four Steps To Owning Your Awkward, the SENSE Framework for offering someone help, the BRAVE Framework for asking for help, The Stress Dispenser, The Exhaustion Funnel, the M-Plan – phew! These are all yours to use, to play with, to be curious about and to make your own. Rather than starting with a blank page, they give you ways to check in with others and, critically, they will help you understand your own mental health and practise the self-care you deserve, which will also help you support others more effectively. Win/Win. Now to use them, practise with them. You've got this.

Communication

The power of the pause, I hope, is one of the most useful take-aways from this book and is both a practical and magical skill you can add to how you communicate. Celebrate the silence, the gift of being quiet and not feeling like you need to immediately talk to fill the gap in a conversation. Remember that someone might be trying to find the words or the courage to talk about their feelings and their mental health and so the greatest gift you can give them is time, space and your attention whilst they find the language and their voice.

The frameworks and conversation starters are also part of your well-stocked communication toolkit because having an immediate jumping-off point for a conversation gives you the freedom to then freestyle, if you wish, perhaps more authentically and meaningfully. Listening means you are holding the space for the other person to use as they need, not how you want, and communicating in one of the most powerful ways by *fully* paying attention. I hope you'll also take from the stories shared here in this book how sometimes the most needed, and often awkward, communication is the one with yourself and how it can bring the greatest change for good.

Compassion

By reading and engaging with this book, right up to here, the last chapter, you are demonstrating the compassion already within you. Reading and connecting with other people's stories and experiences will have deepened your understanding of the human condition, expanding your compassion to even greater levels of generosity and capacity, and remember, the more you give, the more you get back. And gulp, you're getting more comfortable, I hope, with the uncomfortable ideas of self-care and, easy now, self-love, knowing that when we prioritize our own wellbeing, we're topping up our ability to care for others.

HACKING MENTAL HEALTH

In 2019 Nadya Powell and I co-designed a training product called Hacking Mental Health. Fast-track training through some of the fundamentals of understanding mental health and how to talk about it. It's super collaborative, fun to do as a group and a good way to stick your toe in the water of the subject – come do it with me! In the meantime, enjoy the fact that in some ways reading this book is a hack in itself. Ready for more? Become a Mental Health First Aider! Want to take SENSE, BRAVE and Owning Your Awkward further? Join in and learn more at www.ownyourawkward.com.

ALL THE OTHER AWKWARDS

This book is about Owning Your Awkward in order to get comfy having uncomfy conversations about mental health, but think about it, there are plenty of other "awkwards" in our lives aren't there? The principles and tactics found here, especially the Four Steps To Owning Your Awkward, can be applied to topics that can all impact and affect our mental health, from menopause, menstruation and money to midlife, masculinity and mortality – seriously, though, do all awkward topics begin with M?

AWKWARD IS YOUR GREATEST ASSET!

You can do this! You're ready. Confidence? Check! Capability? Yup! Communication? Got it! Compassion? Right here!

Nerves? Present! Hold on, nerves? That wasn't the plan. Relax, nerves are okay; they too are there because you are ready. It's understandable, it's normal. It's because you care and you are ready to put what you've learned into action. Reframe the nerves ... This is a moment to embrace your awkward and ask or act. Your best is better than you think. You have the tools and opportunity to make the greatest difference to someone, or even yourself. Start a conversation. Awkward really is your greatest asset!

AND WHAT NEXT FOR ME?

Life moves forward. I choose small joys over the search for permanent happiness or the manufactured and unrealistic definitions of modern-day "success". I remind myself regularly that help, hope and gratitude are far more important than business deals, balance sheets and, as much as I love it, being bound to my MacBook. As well as using my M-Plan and The Six Supports, I try my best to embrace my daily dos (make the bed, work hard on not working hard, take meds and supplements, stand barefoot on the grass, drink water, family first, look at some art, show gratitude and keep talking) and check that my daily don'ts aren't creeping in (don't over-commit, don't scroll for too long on social media, don't compare and despair, don't take too long to get out of bed, don't hang out with people who make me feel "less than", don't rake over the past, don't worry about the future and don't *ever* believe the hype). Yes, it takes work, and my life is better for it.

Pjoys has *the* most exciting plans afoot, with some of the most loved brands in the world that want to make a difference in partnership with us. Mental Health First Aid England's role in training the nation's workforce is more critical than ever and I'm right there at their side cheerleading the journey. The Own Your Awkward podcast has launched, the book has been written, more talks and more training are coming and more conversations about mental health are being started. And as I dot the i's and cross the t's of this book, Livity is moving into its next phase of life, which most likely means the end of an era for me, and with so much pride, it feels right. Oh yes, and I've just received a diagnosis of a type of ADHD (Attention Deficit Hyperactivity Disorder) – I told you I was a work in progress! But above and beyond all of this, I have love, so much love.

Be Kind

Aside from the awkward rallying cry, I'd like to encourage you to add the mantra of "be kind" alongside your new and improved ability to talk about mental health. Without the kindness of others, help and recovery may never have happened for me and for so many others experiencing poor mental health. By learning to be kind to myself (a lifetime's work), I feel like, maybe, just maybe, I'm becoming a better human with more joy to give and receive. And, today, I'll take that maybe.

Awkward and Awesome

Right now, as I type away, I'm good. Really good! How I'll be tomorrow, goodness knows. Do any of us really know? I do know this – PJ days are okay! And if I need one, I'll take one. As we say at Pjoys … life isn't perfect, it isn't black and white, embrace the *and* in life:

- I am joy *and* pain.
- I am happy *and* sad.
- I have wisdom *and* anxiety.
- I have order *and* chaos.
- I am elegant *and* awkward.
- And I am most certainly brilliant *and* mad.

And in knowing, accepting and embracing all of this, I am more able to be myself than ever before.

- Because without sadness how can I truly know what happiness is?
- Without the pain of my experience, I wouldn't have such gratitude for the joy I now know.
- Without a little bit of madness maybe I'd have never embraced the brilliant moment when I realized I could make mental health an everyday conversation by starting up a pyjamas and being well business.
- Had I not embraced and taken ownership of my awkwardness, I'd have never discovered the elegance and authenticity in helping others own theirs.

And with none of the above I wouldn't have written this book.

I love Owning My Awkward and I hope you love owning yours too.

Meesh x

Mental Health Conditions

Whilst this book is not about learning to become a mental health professional, being equipped with reliable information and knowledge about mental ill-health will set you up more confidently to use the SENSE and BRAVE frameworks with a greater sense of capability and the ability to communicate more comfortably. The descriptions and symptoms can become part of the positive, non-judgemental language you use when you have a conversation about mental health. To understand what someone might be experiencing because you have taken the time to become familiar with different disorders and their symptoms is also, I think, a great act of compassion.

My psychologist, Dr Rumina Taylor, Clinical Psychologist and Chief Clinical Officer, and her team at HelloSelf have provided some accessible explanations of some of the most common mental health disorders and issues, including the symptoms. This section broadly moves from types of mood disorders to anxiety disorders, psychosis and related illnesses, Perinatal Mental Health (PMH) issues, eating disorders and personality disorders.

If you identify with any of the descriptions, disorders and symptoms covered in this chapter and are not already under the care of a mental health professional, please do Own Your Awkward and have a conversation with someone you trust about what you are experiencing. Do seek professional support.

DEPRESSION

Depression (sometimes referred to as clinical depression, major depressive disorder or Dysthymia) is a mood disorder characterized by persistent sadness that lasts for a few weeks or months. Depression can vary in severity and whilst some individuals may only experience one episode of depression in their lifetime, others can experience multiple episodes for extended periods of time.

Although we all may experience fluctuations in our mood, and more specifically short-lived periods of low mood, depression differs from this due to its long-lasting effects. Depression can cause great suffering and can impact multiple aspects of a person's life. There may be difficulties at work, school or with personal relationships. There are many successful treatments available for depression and it's important to find what works best for the individual. By finding the right treatment and support, most people with depression can make a full recovery.

Symptoms
Depression can cause both psychological and physical symptoms, which vary between individuals:
- Low mood or sadness
- Feelings of hopelessness
- Feeling tearful, guilt-ridden or irritable
- Having no or less motivation
- Struggling to enjoy activities that are normally enjoyable
- Finding it difficult to make decisions
- Feeling anxious or worried
- Having suicidal thoughts or thoughts of self-harm

- Moving or speaking more slowly than usual
- Changes in weight or appetite
- Lack of energy
- Loss of sex drive
- Changes to the menstrual cycle
- Disturbed sleep or changes in sleep pattern

ANXIETY DISORDERS

Anxiety is a normal emotion that everyone experiences at times, to a lesser or larger degree. It is a general term for a set of symptoms, physical and psychological, which often is a natural way for our body to respond to threat – real or imagined. Anxiety can become problematic when the response becomes out of proportion with the perceived levels of threat over a regular and escalating period of time.

Symptoms

Regardless of the type of anxiety, there are a few symptoms common to anxiety in general, as listed below:

- Feeling nervous, restless and on edge. Some people have a feeling that something bad is going to happen. There may also be a sensation of butterflies in the stomach that can cause nausea and a loss of appetite.
- Pounding heart – the heart rate may increase.
- Changes to breathing (hyperventilation). Some people start breathing more rapidly.

- More frequent visits to the toilet.
- Shaking and sweating. Trembling hands or trembling all over – it is common to experience shaky legs in addition to increased sweating.
- Difficulty concentrating – struggling to focus on the task at hand, being repeatedly distracted by worrying thoughts or physical sensations.
- Worrying about worrying. Being concerned that stopping worrying will mean things get worse or worrying about the effects of worrying too much.
- Seeking reassurance from others or avoidance of people or places that seem to cause anxiety. These strategies may help in the short-term, but can sometimes maintain and/or exacerbate anxiety in the longer term.
- Fatigue – being in a heightened state of anxiety can be tiring and some people report feeling weak. Sleep can also be disrupted as anxious people find it hard to fall asleep or wake frequently worrying about things.
- Racing thoughts, which can sometimes be repetitive and focus on one specific topic or represent many different areas at once.
- Detachment – feeling distant from the environment or like it's not real.

PANIC ATTACKS

Panic attacks are a fear response and experienced when there is a sudden and rapid increase in anxiety. If someone starts to recognize a set of symptoms specific to their experience of having a panic attack, it can be the first step toward learning how to cope more effectively. Panic attacks usually last no more than ten minutes, and rarely any longer than an hour.

Symptoms

- Symptoms of anxiety (see above).
- Sudden feelings of terror or thoughts of doom. Some people have a feeling something bad is going to happen or that they are about to lose control over the here-and-now.
- Tingling and numbing sensations in the hands, with possibly an urge to clench and unclench the fists.
- Worrying that you will die. While this is understandable given there is often a real physiological effect, panic attacks are not life-threatening.

ACUTE STRESS DISORDER AND POST-TRAUMATIC STRESS DISORDER

Trauma sits within the group of anxiety disorders and describes the psychological effects caused by a distressing or frightening event or series of events. It can develop immediately after experiencing the event, commonly known as Acute Stress Disorder (ASD), or months or even years later, known as Post-Traumatic Stress Disorder (PTSD).

ASD and PTSD can occur in the aftermath of trauma, and trauma can also result in conditions such as depression and anxiety or other mental health difficulties. Examples of the types of events that could cause traumatic reactions include accidents involving injury, bereavement, medical emergencies, violence, natural disasters, war, prolonged bullying, neglect and abuse. Trauma can be caused by experiencing an event directly or indirectly, for example by witnessing something traumatic happening to someone else. ASD and PTSD can have a significant impact on daily functioning and wellbeing and can lead to feelings of isolation, irritability and guilt. Fortunately, whilst the symptoms can be severe and debilitating, there are several evidence-based treatments available.

Symptoms

Whilst the specific symptoms can vary between individuals, symptoms of ASD/PTSD usually fall into the following categories:

- Re-experiencing. A person involuntarily relives the trauma as a flashback, through nightmares, repetitive and distressing images or as a physical sensation (e.g. pain, sweating, trembling). The individual may also experience negative thoughts or questions about the event, which can lead to feelings of anxiety, guilt or shame.
- Avoidance and emotional numbing. Avoidance of reminders of the trauma (e.g. avoiding a person or place that reminds you of the event). Emotional numbing is when an individual may try to deal with their feelings by trying not to feel anything at all. This can lead to isolation and withdrawal from others or activities that previously may have been enjoyed.

- Hyperarousal. An individual may feel easily startled, highly anxious and constantly aware of potential threats, and therefore may find it difficult to relax. Hyperarousal in turn can lead to irritability, feelings of anger, and difficulty sleeping and concentrating.
- Other difficulties. These include other mental health difficulties, such as low mood or motivation, anxiety, phobias, drug or alcohol misuse, self-harming and destructive behaviour. Physical symptoms such as headaches, dizziness, chest pains and stomach aches can also be experienced.

PHOBIAS

We are all born with only two fears: one is the fear of falling and the other the fear of loud noises. Any and all other fears are acquired, adding to our Frame of Reference and that unique Life Footprint we each have (see page 48).

A specific phobia is an overwhelming and debilitating fear of an object, place, situation, feeling or animal. It is not necessarily just something someone is afraid of – the response tends to be more pronounced and can affect how they live their daily life. The response to the phobic stimuli is usually considered to be irrational or exaggerated by observers, but for the individual involved the sense of danger and experience of anxiety can be very distressing and overwhelming. Most people find a simple and isolated phobia is easier to cope with if it is something that can be avoided. However, if a phobia becomes severe it can start to restrict daily functioning or impact on a person's wellbeing, particularly if avoiding the stimuli is causing them to miss out. For example, an individual may feel compelled to turn down a desired job as they are fearful of travelling to work by train.

Symptoms
- Avoidance behaviour
- Panic attacks
- Unsteadiness, dizziness and light-headedness
- Nausea
- Sweating
- Increased heart rate or palpitations
- Shortness of breath
- Trembling or shaking
- An upset stomach
- Fear of losing control
- Fear of fainting
- Feelings of dread
- Fear of dying

OBSESSIVE COMPULSIVE DISORDER

Obsessive Compulsive Disorder (OCD) is characterized by the frequent presence of intrusive thoughts (obsessions) and compulsive behaviours or acts (compulsions). It can be misunderstood and related back to the idea of a person who likes to have things organized. OCD is, in fact, primarily an anxiety disorder characterized by the fear of something bad happening and the person being responsible.

The experience of unwanted and intrusive thoughts causes significant anxiety because of how the thoughts are appraised, which in turn causes compulsive behaviours. For example, if someone is worried that they haven't switched off the oven before leaving the house, they may return home multiple times to check this. The anxiety caused by the fear of accidentally causing damage to themselves or others can be distressing and result in the person feeling compelled to complete checking behaviour to relieve this anxiety.

Symptoms

- Obsession. When an unwanted, intrusive and often distressing thought, image or urge repeatedly enters a person's mind. When this pattern of thinking causes persistent, unpleasant thoughts that start to interrupt the usual train of thought, it starts to become disruptive and distressing for the individual. Common obsessions usually focus around a fear of deliberately or accidentally harming themselves or others, fear of contamination by disease or infection, or a need for symmetry or orderliness.
- Compulsive repetitive behaviours or mental acts. These are behaviours a person feels driven to perform as a result of the anxiety and distress caused by the obsession. Compulsions arise to reduce or prevent the anxiety caused by the obsession. For example, an individual who

fears contamination may repeatedly wash their hands. Most individuals with OCD realize that this behaviour is irrational, but many do it anyway just in case. The compulsive behaviour temporarily can relieve the anxiety, but the obsession and anxiety soon return, causing the cycle to begin again. Some individuals with OCD may only have compulsions or obsessive thoughts, but most will experience both. Examples of compulsive behaviours include:

o Cleaning and handwashing
o Checking
o Counting
o Ordering and arranging
o Hoarding
o Seeking reassurance
o Repeating words in their mind
o Thinking "neutralizing" thoughts to counter the obsessions
o Avoiding places and situations that could trigger obsessions

BODY DYSMORPHIC DISORDER

Body Dysmorphic Disorder (BDD) is a mental health condition, closely related to OCD, where an individual spends a large amount of time worrying about a perceived flaw in their appearance that is often unnoticeable or seen as minor by others. The individual usually spends at least an hour a day (collectively) pre-occupied by this flaw, and can experience intrusive thoughts and engage in repetitive checking behaviours to ease the distress they suffer.

Behaviours may include looking at themselves in reflective surfaces, trying to camouflage, alter or minimize their perceived flaw or avoiding situations that may trigger feelings of anxiety (e.g. social situations where they feel they may be seen and judged by others). BDD is also associated with feelings of shame for the individual and, understandably, can be very distressing to talk about with others for fear of appearing vain or self-obsessed. These behaviours are completed in an attempt to make a person feel better (e.g. camouflaging) or to confirm the belief that they do look as bad as they thought (e.g. checking appearance). However, these behaviours, although reducing anxiety in the short-term, can lead to an increase in preoccupation and distress with appearance.

Symptoms
- Worry and preoccupation about a specific area of the body (particularly the face).
- Time spent comparing appearance with that of other people.
- Increased amounts of time spent looking in the mirror or other shiny surfaces, or avoiding mirrors altogether.
- Attempts to conceal flaws by, for example, combing hair in a particular way, and spending increased amounts of time applying make-up or choosing clothes.
- Picking at skin to make it "smooth".

PSYCHOSIS

Psychosis (also called a "psychotic experience" or "psychotic episode") is when an individual perceives and interprets reality in a different way from people around them. It can be described as "losing touch" with reality. It presents itself in a variety of ways, the most common symptom being hallucinations – when a person sees, hears and feels things that other people don't and delusions, which are beliefs that are not based on reality but feel real to the person experiencing them – e.g. believing they are being followed by secret agents. Cognitive experiences and challenges might also be experienced, such as concentration or memory problems, being unable to understand new information or disorganized thinking and speech. There are different types of psychosis, including Bipolar Disorder, Schizophrenia, Schizoaffective Disorder and Perinatal Psychosis. Alcohol misuse can cause alcohol-induced psychosis as can taking cannabis and other drugs misuse.

Psychosis can be very frightening for the person experiencing the episode and they are more likely to cause harm to themselves, rather than others. Surprisingly, many people experience only one episode in their lives.

Symptoms
- Difficulty concentrating
- Depressed mood
- Sleeping too much or not enough
- Anxiety
- Suspiciousness

- Withdrawal from family and friends
- Emerging unusual beliefs
- Hallucinations
- Delusions
- Disorganized speech
- Suicidal thoughts or actions

BIPOLAR DISORDER

Bipolar Disorder is a condition predominantly affecting mood. People with bipolar disorder tend to experience periods of low mood (also known as depression) and periods of elevated/ high mood (also known as mania). It is, of course, a perfectly healthy part of the human condition to experience a range of moods, but in bipolar disorder moods can swing from an extreme high to an extreme low in a way that affects day-to-day functioning.

Bipolar Disorder has two subtypes: Bipolar I and Bipolar II. Bipolar I is diagnosed when a person has experienced at least one episode of mania that lasts longer than a week; the majority of people (around 90%) will also have periods of depression. Bipolar II is diagnosed when a person has had at least one period of significant depression and at least one period of hypomania (similar to mania but milder).

Changes in mood in Bipolar Disorder can last for several weeks or months at a time and are frequently severe enough to interfere with daily life. Some people, but not all, find that they cycle between these two extremes with periods of "normal" mood between episodes. It is also possible to experience a mixed state when symptoms of both depression and mania are present simultaneously. The symptoms during an episode can also affect energy and activity levels as well as ability to function. Bipolar Disorder is considered to be a lifelong diagnosis, but there are many ways in which people are able to manage their mood. As Bipolar is characterized by changes in mood, the symptoms can vary depending on which mood state is being experienced.

Symptoms

- Feeling sad, hopeless or irritable
- Lacking energy
- Difficulty concentrating and remembering things
- Loss of interest in everyday activities
- Feelings of emptiness or worthlessness
- Feelings of guilt and despair
- Self-doubt
- Lack of appetite
- Difficulty sleeping
- Waking up early
- Suicidal thoughts
- Feeling very happy, elated or overjoyed
- Talking very quickly
- Feeling full of energy
- Feeling self-important
- Feeling full of great new ideas and having important plans
- Being easily distracted
- Being easily irritated or agitated
- Having unusual ideas or seeing and hearing things that other people cannot

- Not being able to sleep or thinking you do not need to
- Not eating
- Doing things that are out of character, such as spending large sums of money on expensive and sometimes unaffordable items
- Making decisions or saying things that are out of character and that others see as being risky or harmful

Other health conditions linked to psychosis include malaria, Parkinson's disease, HIV and AIDS, Alzheimer's disease, syphilis, lupus, Lyme disease, brain tumours, urinary tract infections and hypoglycaemia.

PERINATAL MENTAL HEALTH

Perinatal refers to the period during pregnancy, as well as following birth. Perinatal Mental Health (PMH) difficulties are challenges that affect parents during this period. PMH conditions are very common, affecting around 20% of mothers and 10% of fathers. The most commonly experienced difficulty is Postnatal Depression (PND), also known as Postpartum Depression. This differs from the "baby blues", which is a low or overly emotional mood experienced for 3–10 days after the birth. Usually due to the lack of regular sleep, hormonal changes and the new emotional demands placed on the mother, the baby blues go away on their own.

Other perinatal conditions include Perinatal Anxiety, Perinatal Obsessive Compulsive Disorder, Perinatal Post–Traumatic Stress Disorder and Perinatal Psychosis.

PMH conditions are caused by a variety of factors – extreme sleep deprivation can be a trigger – and are by no means an indication that a person is not right for parenthood. It is completely okay, and common, to struggle, and reaching out for help is by no means a statement that someone can't care for their baby – if anything, it highlights their determination to be their best self during those early days, weeks and years.

It should be noted that PMH struggles affect adoptive parents as well as birthing parents, with 8% experiencing Postnatal Depression.

Symptoms of Postnatal Depression
- Feeling upset and tearful
- Being restless, agitated or irritable
- Feeling empty/emotionally numb
- Unable to enjoy things you usually enjoy
- Hostility/indifference to partner
- Hostility/indifference to the baby
- Anxiety
- Stomach pains
- Pins and needles
- Irregular heartbeat
- Difficulty sleeping
- Feeling unable to relax
- Catastrophizing – imagining the worst in each situation
- Feeling like everyone can see the anxiety
- Worried about losing touch with reality

EATING DISORDERS

Eating disorders are serious mental illnesses that are about feelings, rather than food. The person's behaviour with food may make them feel more able to cope, or may make them feel in control, though they might not be aware of the purpose this behaviour is serving.

Eating disorders can affect people of all ages, genders, ethnicities and backgrounds and include Anorexia, Bulimia, binge-eating and Other Specified Feeding or Eating Disorder (OFSED). People with eating disorders use disordered eating behaviour as a way to cope with difficult situations or feelings. This behaviour can include limiting the amount of food eaten, eating very large quantities of food at once, getting rid of food eaten through unhealthy means (e.g. making themselves sick, misusing laxatives, fasting or excessive exercise), or a combination of these behaviours.

Symptoms

- Weight loss
- Avoidance of certain types of food
- Self-induced vomiting
- Self-induced purging
- Excessive exercise
- Use of appetite suppressants and/or diuretics
- Repeated episodes of eating very large amounts of food in short periods of time
- Periods of starvation
- Person perceives themselves too big or heavy

- Intense fear of weight gain
- Preoccupation with food and eating
- Eating alone
- Eating rapidly
- Feeling disgusted, depressed or guilty about eating
- Feeling out of control about eating
- Eating when not feeling physically hungry

PERSONALITY DISORDERS

Our personality is the characteristic set of thoughts, feelings and behaviours that make us who we are. It guides us to make the decisions that we make and impacts all interactions that we have with others. Personality disorders describe conditions where the aforementioned elements of our personality cause us persistent difficulties in our lives. They represent significant deviations from the way in which a typical individual thinks/feels/behaves in certain situations, particularly in relation to others.

We all have aspects of our personality that can prevent us from, at times, being the people we want to be. Those with personality disorders are not fundamentally different to anyone else, but can sometimes need additional help.

Borderline Personality Disorder (BPD), also known as Emotionally Unstable Personality Disorder (EUPD), is the most common presentation of a personality disorder and can be characterized by the symptoms opposite.

Symptoms

- Fear of abandonment or being left alone. A loved one going away for the weekend or coming home late can cause high levels of anxiety and the individual may take steps to stop them from leaving.
- Self-destructive behaviour and self-harm. An increase in risk-taking behaviour can include engaging in dangerous situations, particularly when upset, such as reckless driving, binge-eating, excessive consumption of alcohol and/or drugs and unsafe sex. Self-harm behaviours or suicidal ideation are also not uncommon.
- Extreme mood swings. Rapid cycling between emotional states is common, often due to reasons that others find perplexing. These mood swings are intense but usually short, passing after hours or even minutes.
- Unstable relationships. Relationships with others can be intense or short-lived and can be difficult to maintain – they can seem either perfect or terrible and nowhere in between.
- Lack of identity. For individuals diagnosed with BPD, it can be difficult to identify a strong sense of self at times. It is not uncommon to switch jobs, friendship groups, values or even religion and sexual identity.
- Paranoia and suspicion. Feeling on edge and suspicious about the motives of others. When stressed this can also lead to feeling disconnected from yourself and the world around you, known as disassociation.

GRIEF AND BEREAVEMENT

Grief is a common emotional response to loss. Although it is not an illness or disorder, it feels important to include as it's another conversation and experience that has stigma attached to it. People often avoid using straight language to talk about death and tend to whisper expressions such as "they passed away". It is important to remember that whilst there are some common patterns and stages to grief, each person's experience is individual and can change over time; there is no right or wrong way to feel and there are no timelines within which a person is expected to feel better. There are well-documented stages of grief – denial, anger, bargaining, depression, acceptance – but it is important to remember that these aren't linear and therefore people may move in and out of them over time. If grief persists and disrupts a person's daily life and their ability to function for a long period of time, it may be a sign of something called "complex grief" and professional help should be sought.

Symptoms

As grief is not an illness, there are no symptoms as such, but there can be common experiences, as listed below:
- Feelings such as sadness, numbness, anger and anxiety
- Tearfulness
- Sleeping difficulties
- Withdrawing from people and activities
- Lacking energy and motivation
- Changes in thinking, such as poor concentration and forgetfulness

Acknowledgements

Thanks and gratitude to:

Remi, for your belief, support, and complete and utter unconditional love for me. I love you.

Lili, for your glorious talent of always making me laugh at just the right moment. I love you so, so much.

Mum, for your constant love, care, and encouragement.

My Splisy, Susie, for your beautiful heart and to Dav and LiLi for your love and lolz.

Dad, for your love and support.

Teddy, for the non-judgement and the licks.

Sues, for your love, energy and unrelenting encouragement, even in the most 'bannoying' of moments. We laugh, we cry and we laugh again once more. Dave would be so proud of you and Pjoys. And to your excellent boys, Tim, Freddie, Billy and Louie – here's to more fun times.

And thank you Louie for the word 'bannoying'!

Lulu, for your love and years of friendship, through good times and bad. So many more good times to come lovely Linds. And to your beautiful family, Rob, Scarlett and Max, love you lovelies.

Simon Blake OBE, for your leadership, cheerleading and compassion. And to all the MHFA England family – a community driven by purpose. Thanks also to Shannon Anderson, CEO, MHFA International.

Scott Pendrey, Poppy Jaman OBE, Geoff McDonald, Simon Albert, Penny Knight and all of the Charity Challenge and HSBC crew, for getting me up the hill (and the next one, and the next). And my Personal Trainer, Alexandra McMillan for getting me trek-fit!

My Publisher, Jo Lal, and everyone at Welbeck Balance, for believing in me and this book, every awkward step of the way. I have loved this experience.

My Editor, Dawn Bates, for taking my thoughts and words and making them make sense. I have learned so much from you.

Beth Bishop for your patience and eye for detail!

My Literary Agent, Millie Hoskins and everyone at United Agents for your experience and support.

Bryan Niederhelm at Gavin de Becker & Associates for our rich conversations – you gave me so much.

Jonny Benjamin for your love and courage, and of course, for introducing me to your fab Dad.

Michael Benjamin for being, well, fab and such an amazing support to me on Pjoys.

Chrissie Nicholson, for sharing the weight and giving me so much inspiration.

Tim, Amanda, Poppy, Violet and Wilde for your love and support you beauties!

Dr. Rumina Taylor and Dr. Az Hakeem for your care and contribution.

John and Pauline Moore, for your unwavering encouragement (and all the tea, toast and taxies!).

My dear Gavin, Ella, Robbie and all at Richard Ward Hair – Truly the best talking therapies and an essential part of my self-care!

ACKNOWLEDGEMENTS

Jan King, for your kindness and generosity.

Sandra Wright for turning my COURAGE to BRAVE and Suze Bowerman for turning the book into the podcast.

Sulaiman Khan and Lucy Hobbs for your guidance on language.

Stephen Knight, Lydia Yadhi, Joanna Santinon, Jez Felwick, Alex Goat, Stephen Woodford, Rebecca Watson, Sarah Shore, Katy Wyatt, Jo Sullivan, Bejay Mulenga, Sara Milne Rowe, Suresh Kara, Nicky Hirst, Cristina Escallon, MadC, Xenz, Tristan Eaton, Augustine Kofie, Preys, David Shillinglaw and Crash One – to each of you, I'm grateful.

The Mindfulness-Based Cognitive Therapy (MBCT) family around the world, especially Marion Furr at The Oxford Mindfulness Centre.

The Livity crew, past and present – my love and thanks to you all. With a special thank you to the leadership team of old: Kate, Cal, Lains, Lianre, Alex, Gav and my business partner Sam.

Ruby Wax for writing *A Mindfulness Guide for the Frazzled*.

Michael Acton Smith for creating the Calm App.

Gavin de Becker for writing *The Gift of Fear*.

Brené Brown for my awkward lightbulb moment.

Every brave individual, in each business, organization and network, who has invited me in to share my story, knowledge and training.

All the contributors to this book. I'm overwhelmed by your generosity and grateful for the value and diversity your stories and voices bring to this book.

References

Åsberg, M. Mindfulness Exhaustion Funnel. Karolinska Institute, Stockholm.

De Becker, G (2000). *The Gift of Fear*. Bloomsbury Publishing.

Chisholm, D et al (2016). Scaling-up treatment of depression and anxiety: a global return on investment analysis. *The Lancet Psychiatry, vol. 3*, no. 5, pp. 415-424. Available at: doi:10.1016/S2215-0366(16)30024-4

Evans-Lacko, S & Knapp, M (2016). Global patterns of workplace productivity for people with depression: absenteeism and presenteeism costs across eight diverse countries. *Social Psychiatry and Psychiatric Epidemiology, vol. 51, no.* 11, pp. 1525–1537. Available at: doi:10.1007/s00127-016-1278-4

Hanh, TN (1993). *Love in Action: Writings on Nonviolent Social Change*. Parallax Press.

Hoey, JK (2017). *Build Your Dream Network: Forging Powerful Relationships in a Hyper-Connected World*. Tarcherperigee.

Holmes, EA et al (2020). Multidisciplinary research priorities for the COVID-19 pandemic: a call for action for mental health science. *Lancet Psychiatry*, vol. 7, pp. 547–60 Available at: doi.org/10.1016/ S2215-0366(20)30168-1

Keyes, CLM (2002). The Mental Health Continuum: From Languishing to Flourishing in Life. *Journal of Health and Social*

Behavior, vol. 43, no. 2, pp. 207–222. Available at: www.jstor.org/stable/3090197

The Lancet (2018). The Global Burden of Diseases, Injuries, and Risk Factors Study 2017. *Global Health Metrics*, vol. 392, no. 10,159, pp. 1789–1858. Available at: doi.org/10.1016/S0140-6736(18)32279-7

International Committee of the Red Cross (2020). World Mental Health Day: New Red Cross survey shows COVID-19 affecting mental health of one in two people. [online] Available at: www.icrc.org/en/document/world-mental-health-day-red-cross-covid-19-mental-health-survey

Mental Health First Aid International. Mental Health is a Global Priority. [online] Available at: mhfainternational.org/mental-health-is-a-global-priority

Mental Health Taskforce NE (2016) . The Five Year Forward View for Mental Health. Available at: england.nhs.uk

O'Shea, N (2020). Forecasting needs and risks in the UK. Centre for Mental Health. [pdf] Available at: www.centreformentalhealth.org.uk/sites/default/files/publication/download/CentreforMentalHealth_COVID_MH_Forecasting3_Oct20_0.pdf

Patel, V et al (2018). The Lancet Commission on global mental health and sustainable development. *The Lancet Commissions*, vol. 392, no. 10,157, pp. 1553–1598. Available at: doi.org/10.1016/S0140-6736(18)31612-X

Schiff, JL, Schiff, A & Schiff, E (1975). Frames of Reference. *Transactional Analysis Bulletin*, vol. 5, no. 3, pp. 290–294. Available at: doi.org/10.1177/036215377500500320

Wax, R (2016). *A Mindfulness Guide for the Frazzled.* Penguin Life.

Williams, M & Penman, D (2011). *Mindfulness: A Practical Guide to Finding Peace in a Frantic World*. Little, Brown Book Group.

World Health Organization (2018). Mental health: strengthening our response. Available at: www.who.int/news-room/fact-sheets/detail/mental-health-strengthening-our-response

World Health Organization (2018). *Mental Health Atlas 2017*. Available at: *www.who.int/publications/i/item/9789241514019*

World Health Organization (2019). Burn-out an "occupational phenomenon": International Classification of Diseases. Available at: https://www.who.int/news/item/28-05-2019-burn-out-an-occupational-phenomenon-international-classification-of-diseases

World Health Organization (2021). Suicide worldwide in 2019: Global Health Estimates. Available at: www.who.int/teams/mental-health-and-substance-use/suicide-data

Useful Resources

UK

In a Crisis
The Samaritans: 116 123; jo@samaritans.org, 24/7 service
Text SHOUT: 85258, 24/7 service

General Resources
ADHD Foundation: www.adhdfoundation.org.uk
Anxiety UK: www.anxietyuk.org.uk
Best Beginnings: www.bestbeginnings.org.uk
Black African and Asian Therapy Network: www.baatn.org.uk
Black Minds Matter: www.blackmindsmatteruk.com
Campaign Against Living Miserably (CALM):
www.thecalmzone.net
Heads Together: www.headstogether.org.uk
HelloSelf: www.helloself.com
Hub of Hope: www.hubofhope.co.uk
The Institute for Muslim Mental Health:
www.muslimmentalhealth.com/islam-mental-health
Mental Health Foundation UK: www.mentalhealth.org.uk
MHFA England: www.mhfaengland.org
Mind UK: www.mind.org.uk

No More Panic: www.nomorepanic.co.uk
No Panic: www.nopanic.org.uk
Papyrus: www.papyrus-uk.org
Rethink Mental Illness: www.rethink.org
Scope: www.scope.org.uk
Scottish Association for Mental Health (SAMH): www.samh.org.uk
Social Anxiety: www.social-anxiety.org.uk
Stonewall: www.stonewall.org.uk
Young Minds: www.youngminds.org.uk

EUROPE

Mental Health Europe: www.mhe-sme.org
Mental Health Ireland: www.mentalhealthireland.ie

USA

In a Crisis

Suicide Prevention Lifeline: www.suicidepreventionlifeline.org; 1-800-273-8255, 24/7 service

General Resources

American Foundation for Suicide Prevention: afsp.org
Anxiety and Depression Association of America: www.adaa.org
HelpGuide: www.helpguide.org
Mental Health America: www.mhanational.org
Mentalhealth.gov: www.mentalhealth.gov

MHFA USA: www.mentalhealthfirstaid.org
National Alliance on Mental Illness (NAMI): www.nami.org
National Institute of Mental Health: www.nimh.nih.gov
Very Well Mind: www.verywellmind.com

CANADA

In a Crisis

Canada Suicide Prevention Service: www.crisisservicescanada.ca;
1-833-456-4566, 24/7 service; text 45645, 4pm–midnight

General Resources

Anxiety Canada: www.anxietycanada.com
Canadian Association for Suicide Prevention:
www.suicideprevention.ca
Canadian Mental Health Association: cmha.ca
Crisis Service Canada: www.ementalhealth.ca
MHFA Canada: www.mhfa.ca

AUSTRALIA AND NEW ZEALAND

In a Crisis

Lifeline: 131114, 24/7 service; text 0477 13 11 14, noon–midnight

General Resources

Anxiety New Zealand Trust: www.anxiety.org.nz

Beyond Blue: www.beyondblue.org.au

Embrace Multicultural Mental Health: www.embracementalhealth.org.au

Head to Health: headtohealth.gov.au

Health Direct: www.healthdirect.gov.au

Lifelife: www.lifeline.org.au

Mental Health Australia: mhaustralia.org

Mental Health Foundation of New Zealand: www.mentalhealth.org.nz

MHFA Australia: www.mhfa.com.au

SANE Australia: www.sane.org

TriggerHub.org is one of the most elite and scientifically proven forms of mental health intervention

Trigger Publishing is the leading independent mental health and wellbeing publisher in the UK and US. Clinical and scientific research conducted by assistant professor Dr Kristin Kosyluk and her highly acclaimed team in the Department of Mental Health Law & Policy at the University of South Florida (USF), as well as complementary research by her peers across the US, has independently verified the power of lived experience as a core component in achieving mental health prosperity. Specifically, the lived experiences contained within our bibliotherapeutic books are intrinsic elements in reducing stigma, making those with poor mental health feel less alone, providing the privacy they need to heal, ensuring they know the essential steps to kick-start their own journeys to recovery, and providing hope and inspiration when they need it most.

Delivered through TriggerHub, our unique online portal and accompanying smartphone app, we make our library of bibliotherapeutic titles and other vital resources accessible to individuals and organizations anywhere, at any time and with complete privacy, a crucial element of recovery. As such, TriggerHub is the primary recommendation across the UK and US for the delivery of lived experiences.

At Trigger Publishing and TriggerHub, we proudly lead the way in making the unseen become seen. We are dedicated to humanizing mental health, breaking stigma and challenging outdated societal values to create real action and impact. Find out more about our world-leading work with lived experience and bibliotherapy via triggerhub. org, or by joining us on:

🐦 @triggerhub_

📘 @triggerhub.org

📷 @triggerhub_

Printed in the USA
CPSIA information can be obtained
at www.ICGtesting.com
JSHW031708140824
68134JS00038B/3584